HEALTHY

SLEEP

HABITS,

HAPPY

TWINS

*A step-by-step programme for
a good night's sleep*

Dr Marc Weissbluth

Vermilion
LONDON

1 3 5 7 9 10 8 6 4 2

Published in 2010 by Vermilion, an imprint of Ebury Publishing
First published in the USA by Ballantine Books, an imprint of The Random House
Publishing Group, a division of Random House, Inc., New York, in 2009

Ebury publishing is a Random House Group Company

The Random House Group Limited Reg. No. 954009

Addresses for companies within the Random House Group can be found at
www.rbooks.co.uk

A CIP catalogue record for this book is available from the British Library

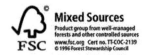

Mixed Sources
Product group from well-managed
forests and other controlled sources
www.fsc.org Cert no. TT-COC-2139
© 1996 Forest Stewardship Council
FSC

The Random House Group Limited supports The Forest Stewardship
Council (FSC), the leading international forest certification organisation. All our
titles that are printed on Greenpeace approved FSC certified paper carry the FSC logo.
Our paper procurement policy can be found at www.rbooks.co.uk/environment

Printed in the UK by CPI Mackays, Chatham, ME5 8TD

Book design by Jo Anne Metsch

ISBN 9780091935207

Copies are available at special rates for bulk orders.
Contact the sales development team on 020 7840 8487 for more information.

To buy books by your favourite authors and register for offers, visit www.rbooks.co.uk

Please note that conversions to imperial weights and measures
are suitable equivalents and not exact.

The information in this book has been compiled by way of general guidance in relation to
the specific subjects addressed, but is not a substitute and not to be relied on for medical,
healthcare, pharmaceutical or other professional advice on specific circumstances and in
specific locations. Please consult your GP before changing, stopping or starting any medical
treatment. So far as the author is aware the information given is correct and up to date as
at May 2009. Practice, laws and regulations all change, and the reader should obtain up-to-
date professional advice on any such issues. The author and publishers disclaim, as far as
the law allows, any liability arising directly or indirectly from the use, or misuse, of
the information contained in this book.

This book is dedicated,

with all my love, to Linda

Contents

Introduction / *ix*

PART I
UNDERSTANDING SLEEP IN CHILDREN / *1*

CHAPTER 1
The Importance of Sleep for the Whole Family / *3*

CHAPTER 2
What Is Healthy Sleep? / *16*

PART II
SLEEP STRATEGIES FOR TWINS
AND MULTIPLES / *33*

CHAPTER 3
How to Sleep-Train Twins / *35*

CHAPTER 4
Creating a Sleep-Training Team / *66*

CHAPTER 5

Children's Sleep Needs at Different Ages / *85*

PART III

TROUBLESHOOTING / *121*

CHAPTER 6

Breastfeeding Twins: Special Challenges,
Special Tips / *123*

CHAPTER 7

Anticipating and Preparing for Possible
Challenges with Sleep Training / *139*

Resources / *155*

Acknowledgements / *161*

Index / *163*

Introduction

Congratulations on your twins or multiples! Twins and multiples are more than double the fun: this is an exciting and magical time for your growing family.

Whether you're still expecting and are reading this book to prepare for life with your new babies or have already brought the babies home from the hospital and are starting to feel the effects of sleep deprivation, I hope this book will help you enjoy your babies more and be less anxious about their needs. Read front to back or in fits and starts, this book will give you the information you need to help your children begin to fall asleep on their own, stay asleep, and sleep regularly. Which means that in a short time, the whole family – Mum and Dad included – will be more rested and generally happier.

As founder of the original Sleep Disorders Center at Children's Memorial Hospital in Chicago, USA, I have studied both healthy and disturbed sleep in thousands of children. I have also been a paediatrician for more than thirty-five years and am the father of four children (and six grandchildren, at this writing). It is this combined experience that helped me develop the method I call 'sleep training', a process for instituting a daily routine and teaching infants to soothe themselves. My first book, *Healthy Sleep Habits, Happy Child,* details the sleep-training technique for children of all ages and, I'm proud to say, has helped almost a million families get a better night's sleep.

More recently, I conducted an interesting research project with the parents of twins whom I met through my practice or in twin support groups that I've conducted through the years. I had more than a hundred sets of parents fill out an extensive survey so that I could better understand their experience with sleep-training their twins, their concerns and their questions. I heard countless stories of how getting twins to sleep well and sleep on a schedule was clearly worth the effort. Mothers who were getting more sleep themselves reported less baby blues and postpartum depression. Mothers also told me that getting their babies to sleep well made them generally less anxious about taking care of their twins: feeds got easier, and everyone's mood was improved. Fathers also reported much less tension – in their wives, in themselves and in their marriages. The answers and comments these parents provided has largely guided the information I will share in this book.

Sleep-training twins presents special challenges. The fundamental issue is obviously that there is not enough of you to go around most of the time! With one baby, mothers and fathers (and their help, if they choose to get it) can take turns feeding and caring for that baby during the day and during the night so that, in theory at least, one of the parents is rested most of the time. With twins, either one parent is pulling double duty or both parents are sharing the load the best way they can work out. Either way, parents of twins often wish they could clone themselves so that they could both get more of a break from the seemingly endless rush to soothe, feed, change or – happily – play with the twins. Without this futuristic technology, this book offers special solutions for sleep-training your multiples. I offer help for bleary-eyed parents – sleep and some semblance of a routine will return to your family soon!

Beyond giving me a better understanding of the unique challenges involved in getting twins and multiples to sleep, my recent research also revealed some interesting facts about sleep patterns in twins. Parents report that fraternal twins are harder to get to sleep because they are often fundamentally not on the same 'clock' or schedule. Identical twins seem to be more in sync with each other from the very start, and many parents of identical twins find that they have an easier time getting the twins to be on the same sleep schedule.

My research also revealed some interesting results about the ways in which parental age and experience impact sleep-training twins. Some older parents reported feeling that their age was an advantage because they felt it gave them the benefit of more confidence, patience and tolerance for the crying that sometimes accompanies sleep training. Other older parents felt that their age was a factor in their exhaustion and were therefore highly motivated to sleep-train their twins as soon as possible.

Whether or not Mum underwent assisted reproductive technology (ART) to conceive her twins also seems to indirectly impact the babies' sleep. Some mums who underwent protracted ART efforts reported having very little motivation to impose schedules or sleep training on their twins; instead, they wanted to spend as much waking time as possible with their twins and wanted to soothe their children to sleep at the breast or by holding and rocking them instead of teaching them self-soothing techniques. Mothers in my survey who reported experiencing baby blues or postpartum depression had a harder time sleep-training their twins, likely because they were having an all-around harder time with the transition to motherhood. That said, sleep training – and the rest for everyone that comes with it – turned out to be one of the things that greatly helped lift their depression. Chapter 7 outlines and summarises my survey findings so that you can anticipate and prepare for the possibility of having a similar experience.

Even knowing these trends, however, what's important to take away from the results of my study is that sleep training can work and work well – quickly – for twins, whether fraternal or identical, conceived using ART or otherwise! Indeed, the process of falling asleep is learned behaviour. I will do my best to make sure that you find a comfortable way to teach your twins how to become great sleepers.

A word about how to use this book: Part I gives you the fundamentals of sleep – why we all need it and what 'healthy' sleep comprises. Many people say, 'What's not to understand? I need sleep, my babies need sleep, tell me how to get it!' and I certainly understand the impulse to skip this descriptive section and get on with the business of learning to sleep-train your children. But I hope that even if you skip ahead to 'Sleep Strategies for Twins and Multiples' (Part II) or 'Troubleshooting' (Part III), you will eventually circle back and read Part I as well. I can't underscore enough the importance of understanding sleep fundamentals. With a greater appreciation of what goes into 'good' or healthy sleep, you may become more motivated to provide it for your children.

Last but not least, I want to point out that throughout this book you will periodically find the comments of parents of multiples that I have worked with or studied. I hope you will find some comfort in hearing about their experiences. I find that in just sharing their frustrations and their successes, new parents can teach one another so much.

The goal of this book is a well-rested family. Happy and healthy sleep to you!

DR MARC WEISSBLUTH

PART I

Understanding Sleep in Children

CHAPTER 1

The Importance of Sleep for the Whole Family

There's nothing like a good night's sleep to help us cope with the challenges of each new day. Most of us define 'good sleep' as having to do with the duration and the depth of rest we get; it's about both quantity and quality. There is actually more that goes into the definition of 'good sleep', and that is the subject of chapter 2. For the moment, I want to turn your attention more generally to *why* sleep matters so much.

The expression 'sleep like a baby' refers to that deep, peaceful sleep that we observe in babies. But as parents of most infants know, it's often the case that those charmingly serene little sleepers can pop awake and stay awake and can also have a terrible time getting to their needed slumber in the first place.

'Needed' is the operative word here; babies need quality sleep, and when they don't get enough of it, everything is off, including their ability to get to sleep again. This might not make much immediate sense to you; many parents think that tiring a baby out over the course of a day will help him sleep better at night. Indeed, the single most common misconception is that babies will simply sleep when they are tired and if they are kept up longer, they will sleep better.

As we'll discuss below, the opposite is true. Babies who are even a little overtired will have a more difficult time making up that lost sleep or napping on cue.

Skip ahead to Part II if you're ready to get started learning to sleep-train right away, and look to chapter 5 for information about how much sleep is enough in twins of varying ages. But after all that, do come back to this discussion. Having a good understanding of how to get good sleep and what happens when children don't will help you appreciate what your children are going through and may help you understand why they cry so hard when they don't get enough rest.

A LITTLE TIRED IS LIKE A LITTLE SICK

Have you ever been a little sick or injured? Imagine that you have an ordinary cold with low-grade fever, sneezing, runny nose, headache and a cough. After a few days the fever is gone, your nose is less stuffy and the cough is less persistent. But you still feel a little weak and tired from having been sick for a few days. Even though you are ready to get back to your routine and your life, you feel uncomfortable and not at your personal best. Maybe you are a little less playful, less creative, less able to multitask. Maybe you're a little more irritable as well. Being a little tired leaves you in the same predicament. If you've not had a good night's sleep, you won't be able to operate at 100 per cent the next day. Each subsequent night of restlessness or interrupted sleep only compounds the problem. We get crankier and crankier; we may even start to have physical pain (headaches, body aches and such).

So it goes for children as well. When babies and children don't get enough sleep, they are not able to cope as well with what the day brings, and they are less able to take restorative naps during the day or fall into deep sleep quickly the following night. They may also have trouble staying focused on eating when you nurse or bottle-feed them. Of course, because they can't communicate their distress any other way for the time being, they cry. All of this understandably makes parents stressed, but not everyone understands that lack of good sleep is the underlying problem.

We often attribute a baby's crying and discomfort to wind, teething or that dreaded but universal time of the day – the early evening – known to veteran parents as the 'witching hour'. Other times we label our children 'high-spirited' or 'needy', but, actually, it's usually impaired sleep that makes babies fussy, less adaptable, more intense and more frightened in the first place. You might notice these changes more near the end of the day, when their sleep tank nears empty.

Of course, everyone knows that when you are horribly sleep-deprived, you feel bad. But few people realise how even a little sleep loss impairs children's mood and performance.

In our ever-busy lives as adults, sometimes sleep is the last thing on the to-do list. But to put it simply, sleep is not a luxury; it is a biological necessity. We should protect our own adult sleep so that we can think clearly in the short term and for the benefit of our long-term health. We need to nurture and protect our children's sleep for both their present-day comfort and their long-term health as well. Helping your twins learn to soothe themselves, to fall asleep on their own and to stay asleep for restorative periods of time is the key to making sure *everyone* in the family gets the sleep he or she needs!

> **Simply put: sleep is not a luxury; it is a biological necessity!**

HOW SLEEP DEPRIVATION AFFECTS YOU

My research with parents of twins confirms what I have observed as a paediatrician for more than thirty-five years: regardless of how old you are or what you went through to conceive your twins, or whether you have fraternal or identical twins, when they do not sleep well, the primary caregiver – usually Mum – suffers. Sleep deprivation undermines all aspects of her life and interferes with her ability to discover and execute solutions to help the twins sleep better. Ideally, you'll want to talk about sleep solutions before the twins are born, but if you already have them and are already sleep-deprived, get Dad involved in working out the solution.

In addition to the lack of physical coordination, headaches and even gastrointestinal issues that are associated with physical exhaustion, mental stress from sleep deprivation is likely to cause an increased heart rate, a rise in blood pressure, muscular tension, irritability and depression. The physical and mental strain might resemble or trigger baby blues or postpartum depression and can create a severe strain on your marriage. One mother in my survey reported that because she and her husband were so tired, they began to fight, and, at the height of their sleep deprivation, they 'hated each other at night'.

Of course, we do not know whether exhaustion and stress from sleep deprivation mimics, worsens or causes baby blues or postpartum depression. Maybe all three events can occur. What we do know is that sleep deprivation colours one's outlook (the world looks like a darker, more lonely and more difficult place to navigate), exacerbates relationship tensions and makes life generally harder for everyone in the house.

'I remember being so tired at various points that I felt my eyes closing while I was on the phone, midsentence. I was incapable of deciding what to eat. I remember thinking, "I have to hire a maternity nurse, but how can I interview nurses when I'm this knackered?" I threatened to divorce my husband if he didn't return some baby gifts at the exact moment I demanded. I cried every day. I swore I heard the babies crying when I was in the shower, and jumped out of the tub to check on them, to find them sleeping or sitting quietly in their bouncy seats. I under- or overreacted all the

time. I chalk some of this up to hormones, but much of it was also sheer sleep deprivation.'

'At around four to five months the girls began to need more and more soothing and to get less and less sleep. The complete lack of any evening time to eat or speak to my husband (as we often sat in separate darkened rooms, each rocking a baby) made me feel that my life had been entirely consumed by the babies. It did not feel like I had a life. I describe the process of following your sleep-training guidelines as "getting my life back".'

In a sleep-deprived state it's hard enough to meet your own needs (possibly including recovering from a C-section), let alone the needs of two or more babies and a household to boot. Added to this mix are the parental worries surrounding experiences more common to multiples – prematurity, colic or gastrointestinal oesophageal reflux disorder (GORD). See the Resources section for information about these special circumstances.

'I always reference the directions we get on an airline. Put your oxygen mask on, and then assist your child. You are no good to them if you are weak, in pain, tired or impatient. You must give them your calm and consistency. Above all, your love. If you are mentally or physically absent, they suffer. It is your job to take care of yourself, and your sanity will be intact.'

HEALTHY SLEEP IS LIKE HEALTHY FOOD

Consider the similarities between food and sleep. Let's first think about food and food quality. Food is a biological need. Food is energy for the body. Poor-quality food – junk food – damages the body by causing all manner of medical issues, including malnutrition, anaemia, diabetes, heart disease and obesity. A little junk food is okay; a lot is not.

Now let's think about sleep and sleep quality. Sleep is also a biological need. Sleep is energy for the brain; poor-quality sleep harms the brain. Think of poor-quality sleep as junk sleep. Junk sleep is just as bad for our children as is junk food.

Junk sleep causes:

- Exhaustion, and we all know what that feels like!
- Impaired mood. Children become more irritable, angry and easily upset; later on, junk sleep can cause or exacerbate depression in adolescents.
- Impaired social and academic performance. Kids who are lacking sleep will be more hyperactive, oppositional and aggressive.
- Impaired cognitive development. Sleep incorporates learning into permanent memory, causes memory con-solidation, and enhances organisational skills, planning, multitasking and executive functioning.
- Impaired personality. Children become fussy, more in-tense, more frightened and less adaptable.
- Impaired hand-eye coordination (which impacts a whole host of functions, such as athletic performance and fine motor skills).

- Systemic inflammation, increased blood pressure, increased stress hormones.
- Impaired glucose control, which is a factor in diabetes and obesity.

SLEEP AND BRAIN DEVELOPMENT

Dr Christian Guilleminault, who along with Dr William C Dement was the founding editor of *Sleep*, the world's leading journal of sleep research, taught me to consider five fundamental principles of understanding sleep:

1. The sleeping brain is not a resting brain.
2. The sleeping brain functions in a manner different from that of the waking brain.
3. The activity and work of the sleeping brain are purposeful.
4. The process of falling asleep is learned.
5. Providing the growing brain with sufficient sleep is necessary for the ability to concentrate and an easier temperament.

Sleep is the power source that keeps your mind alert and calm. Every night and at every nap, sleep recharges the brain's battery. Unlike a lightbulb, which shuts down completely when it is turned off, your child's sleeping brain is active and purposeful. Providing your child's growing brain with quality sleep is necessary for its development. Sleeping well increases brainpower just as weight lifting strengthens muscles. Sleeping well makes your child physically relaxed and mentally alert; he is at his personal best.

There is one significant difference between muscle strength and brain strength, however. Our resting muscles recover strength during relaxed wakefulness; not so our brains. Unlike other organs, the brain does not recover when resting and awake. Even when you are lying relaxed but awake, in a dark, silent room, the brain remains in a state of quiet readiness, prepared to respond immediately. Quiet, wakeful rest can be refreshing in the short term, but it is not a substitute for sleep. Only sleep restores strength to the brain.

Sleep problems not only disrupt a child's nights, they disrupt his days too, by making him less mentally alert, more inattentive, unable to concentrate and easily distracted. They also make him more physically impulsive, hyperactive or lazy.

When children learn to sleep well, they learn to maintain optimal wakefulness. The notion of optimal wakefulness, also called optimal alertness, is important because we tend to think simplistically of being either awake or asleep. Just as our twenty-four-hour cycle consists of more than just the two states called daytime and nighttime – for instance, dawn and dusk – there are gradations in sleep and wakefulness as well. In sleep, the levels vary from deep sleep to partial arousal; in wakefulness, the levels vary from being wide awake to being groggy.

The importance of optimal wakefulness cannot be overemphasised. If your children do not get all the sleep they need, they may seem either drowsy or hyperalert. If either state lasts for a long time, the results are the same: children with difficult moods and hard-to-control behaviour, certainly not children who are ready and able to enjoy themselves or get the most out of the myriad learning experiences placed before them.

> **Sleep energises the brain. Sleep is the power source that keeps the mind alert and calm. Every night and at every nap, sleep recharges the brain's battery.**

SLEEP BEGETS SLEEP

Young children need naps to remain well rested. Naps help refuel a baby's strength during the day. When they don't nap, as many parents know, infants actually sleep less well when night falls. Here's why: when your child naps, his or her cortisol levels fall, and this reduces stress and makes your child calmer. The calmer he or she is, the easier it is to fall asleep and stay asleep. In other words, sleep begets sleep.

In contrast, think of what happens when you don't get enough sleep. Your body produces stimulating hormones and chemicals to fight the fatigue of sleep deprivation, and you get keyed up. The sympathetic nervous system revs up. You feel a little tense, nervous, excited, jumpy, hyper, edgy, jittery, anxious or wound up tight. Even though you might not want or need it, you get a second wind.

This second wind is designed to combat the fatigue of sleep loss. This burst of energy was important for primitive man to survive. It enabled him to hunt longer, fight harder and flee faster from predators. It's like a turbocharger kicking in. But this heightened state of neurological arousal interferes with falling asleep, and it also interferes with learning. Think of the restless child in school, unable to sit still, fidgeting all the time because he is drowsy from junk sleep, and fighting sleepiness to stay awake.

Of course, if you push yourself too hard and sleep too little, you will eventually crash and sleep. Our babies and children will also collapse exhausted if they are pushed too hard (kept up too long). But the burst of nervous stimulation, the second wind, if it lasts too long, is not healthy for any of us, including our children. It's like driving your car past the red line on your turbocharger for too long a time; the engine is going to break.

When your twins get the sleep they really need – both during the day and at night – they will be in a state of optimal alertness, neither chronically drowsy nor keyed up. In turn they will have an easier time falling asleep again.

TWINS ARE INDIVIDUALS

As I said above, fraternal twins tend to be less in sync with each other than identical twins from the very start, and this can sometimes make sleep-training fraternal twins harder. But it's important to remember that every baby is unique and that twins are first and foremost two separate individuals; in many respects they will likely be quite different. Many parents of twins say that they can see differences in temperament, for instance, very early on.

Every baby is born with individual traits that affect the

amount of physical activity, the duration of sleep and the length of period of crying they will sustain. But all babies differ in more subtle ways. Some are easier to 'read'; they seem to have predictable schedules for feeding and sleeping. These babies also tend to cry less and sleep more. They are better able to self-soothe; they fall asleep more easily; and when they awaken at night they are better able to return to sleep unassisted. But don't blame yourself if one (or both) of your twins cries a lot and is less self-soothing. It's only luck, although social customs may affect how you feel about it.

In societies where the mother holds her babies close all the time and her breasts are always available for nursing and soothing, there are still great differences among siblings in terms of fussiness and crying. To the extent she can, with more than one baby to contend with at a time, Mum usually compensates by increasing the amount of rhythmic, rocking motions or nursing. Or she'll bring one of the babies – or both – into her bed. This is not necessarily good or bad. There are no universally 'right' or 'wrong' ways or 'natural' versus 'unnatural' styles of caring for and raising children.

Fraternal or identical, two boys, two girls, or one (or more) of each, the key to helping your multiples have good sleep for life is to start the sleep-training process early. When you start early, there will be no long bouts of crying and no problems with sleeping down the line. The process of falling asleep unassisted is a skill, and, as with any other skill, it is easier to teach good habits first than it is to correct bad habits later. Also, as with any other skill, success comes only after a period of practice.

There are clearly a great number of reasons to help your young twins get the sleep they need, but before we get into the nuts and bolts of sleep training, it's important that you understand the definition of healthy sleep. That is the topic of the next chapter.

If you start early with sleep training, you will be well along the path to preventing sleep problems in your twins.

CHAPTER 2

What Is Healthy Sleep?

Healthy sleep – the kind that keeps us all mentally nimble and alert and that is important for the growing bodies and brains of our children – is made up of five key elements. Children of different ages need more or less of these components as they grow (and we'll discuss the needs of several age groups throughout this chapter), but when these five elements are in proper balance, children get the rest they need.

1. Sleep duration: night and day
2. Naps
3. Sleep consolidation
4. Sleep schedules and timing of sleep
5. Sleep regularity

As your babies' brains mature, the patterns and rhythms of sleep change as well. If you always adapt your parenting practices to these changes, your children will sleep well.

Parents who do not see these changes or make these adjustments have babies who become overtired.

Though I would discourage you from *counting on* the following changes, there are five turning points in the sleep maturation process for full-term babies that you need to understand. When considering these turning points for your twins, use their due date – not their delivery date – as the starting point, but also only as a general guide. Remember, every baby is different, and if your twins don't hit these marks (or if one doesn't), it is not cause for alarm. Still, be on the lookout for changes to occur at approximately these points:

1. Six weeks, the point at which night sleep starts to lengthen and bedtime starts to drift earlier
2. Twelve to sixteen weeks, during which time daytime sleep starts to regularise and bedtime is earlier
3. Nine months, when night waking for feeding as well as a third daytime nap usually disappear
4. Twelve to twenty-one months, when a morning nap usually disappears from the schedule
5. Three to four years, when the remaining afternoon nap becomes more uncommon

The biological development causing all these changes is under the control of two regulatory mechanisms. Understanding these controlling mechanisms will help you organise your thoughts and plan your actions to ensure healthy sleep for your twins.

The first regulatory system controls the body's need for sleep and has been called the 'homeostatic control mechanism'. In a nutshell, this mechanism accounts for the fact that the longer you go without sleep, the more intense your sleepiness and the more you will search for sleep. If you lose sleep, the body tries to restore it. Going without enough sleep causes sleep pressure to build up and forces you to pay back your sleep debt. This automatic process reflects an internal biological mechanism that we do not control. It is similar to the body wanting to control its temperature; when we get hot, we automatically sweat (assuming we are properly hydrated). Unfortunately, our babies' biological need for sleep is always changing, so we have to be on our toes in order not to miss shifts in sleeping requirements.

The second regulatory system is the 'circadian timing system', sometimes also called the 'internal timing system', and is a dedicated regulatory programme that switches specific genes on and off in response to the light-dark cycle. This mechanism automatically tries to ensure that the body is sleeping at the right time and that when you are asleep, the timing and amounts of different stages and types of sleep are correct. The pattern of these signals changes over weeks, months and years as our babies grow into adults. The pace of these changes is especially quick during the first several months, so it is easy for parents to get a little off tempo. Just when you think you have figured out when your babies need to nap or be put to bed at night, the times change!

SLEEP DURATION: NIGHT AND DAY

Duration is an obvious component of healthy sleep: if you don't sleep long enough you feel tired. But how much sleep is enough? And how can you tell if *your* children are getting enough sleep?

Under three or four months of age (from the due date), an infant's sleep patterns seem mostly to reflect the development of the brain. During these first few weeks, in fact, sleep durations equal sleep needs, since infants' behaviour and sleep durations are influenced mostly by biological factors. But after about three or four months, and perhaps even as early as six weeks, parenting practices can influence sleep duration and, consequently, behaviour.

Chapter 5 will give you more information about how much sleep to expect of your twins at various ages, but there are several things to note about newborns and young infants in general.

During their first few days, newborns sleep about sixteen to seventeen hours total each day, although their longest single sleep period may not be long. It makes no difference whether your twins are breastfed or bottle-fed or whether they are boys or girls.

Between one week and four months, the total daily sleep duration will drift down from sixteen and a half to fifteen hours, while the longest single sleep period – usually during the night – increases by anywhere from four to nine hours. This development of longer sleep periods regularly occurring at night begins at about six weeks post-due date. We know from several studies that this development reflects neurological maturation and is *not* related to the start of feeding solid foods.

Unfortunately, some babies under the age of four months sleep much more and others much less. During the first few months, you can usually assume that your babies are getting sufficient sleep because their internal mechanisms are seeing to it. But if one or both of them cries too much or has extreme fussiness or colic, you might need to assist Mother Nature. See page 56 for techniques to reduce bedtime crying or look to the Resources section on page 155 for resources to help you deal with colic and GORD.

Young infants are very portable. You can take them any-where you want, and when they need to sleep, they will. After about six weeks of age, most babies will become more so-cially aware of people and things around them; after about four months of age, your twins will become interested in barking dogs, wind in the trees and many other curious things, all of which can and will likely disturb their sleep.

For most infants, the time they first make a socially re-sponsive smile (usually at about six weeks post-due date) is when social curiosity or social learning begins. However, under about three or four months of age, most infants are not much disturbed by their environment when it comes to sleeping. When their bodies tell them it is time to sleep, they sleep. When their bodies tell them it is time to wake up, they wake up – even when it is inconvenient for their parents! This is true whether they are fed on demand or according to a regular schedule. Hunger, in fact, seems to have little to do with how babies sleep. A much more likely candidate for influencing a baby's sleeping patterns is the hormone melatonin, which is produced by the baby's brain beginning at about three or four months. This hormone surges at night and has the capability to both induce drowsiness and relax the smooth muscles encircling the gut.

This is why at about three or four months of age day/night confusion and apparent abdominal cramps (colic) begin to disappear.

Furthermore, infants raised in an environment where the lights are constantly on evolve normal sleep patterns, just like babies brought up in homes where the lights are routinely turned on and off. Prematurity – a common occurrence with twins and multiples – doesn't change this equation. Twins born four weeks before their due date, for example, reach the same level of sleep development as a full-term baby four weeks *later* than the child born on time. Biological sleep/wake development does not speed up in 'preemies' who are exposed to more social stimulation.

The Meaning of 'Sleeping Through the Night'

After the first few weeks of life, counting from the due date, you might feed your twins at bedtime between 9 and 11pm and not feed again until 4 or 5am. Is this 'sleeping through the night'?

Perhaps the more helpful term and thing to aim for is 'organised night sleep'. When your twins have a long block of uninterrupted sleep lasting four to six hours, usually occurring before midnight, you can make this claim. This usually starts to happen at about or just past six weeks (counting from their expected due date). At this age, they are falling asleep earlier, between 6 and 8pm, and might need to be fed once or twice

overnight before they get up to start the day around 6 or 7am. You might be lucky and not have to feed them at all overnight, but this is uncommon.

Feeding babies once or twice at night or feeding more often in a family bed is common for the first few months of life, so I personally think you can claim bragging rights for 'sleeping through the night' when they are sleeping well overnight with only one or two feeds.

NAPS

We have all experienced drowsiness in the midafternoon, and when we are able to, this is the time when we take a nap. All adults have a dip in mental alertness at this time because this is a biological rhythm. This sensation of sleepiness is partially – but only partially – related to how long you have been up that day and how long you slept the night before. Nap rhythms are part of our individual makeup.

Naps are an essential component of healthy sleep for young children. The sleep rhythms for daytime sleep in children develop around three to four months of age. I believe that naps that occur at the right time and are sufficiently long lead to optimal daytime alertness for learning – that is, naps adjust the alert/drowsy control to just the right setting for optimal daytime arousal. Without naps, your children will be too drowsy or too distractable to learn well.

In children, a morning nap develops before an afternoon nap, but it also disappears before the afternoon nap. There is more rapid eye movement (REM) sleep or active sleep than quiet sleep in the morning nap. This pattern is reversed in the afternoon nap. Research suggests that high amounts of REM sleep, under the influence of low melatonin levels, help direct the course of brain maturation in early life. Also, adult studies suggest that REM sleep is especially important for restoring us emotionally or psychologically, while deep, non-REM sleep appears to be more important for physical restoration. Let's get all the REM sleep we can for our babies!

As previously mentioned, levels of cortisol, a hormone associated with stress, dramatically fall during a nap, indicating a reduction of stress in the body. Not taking a needed nap means that the body remains stressed.

My studies show that at four months of age, most children take two or three naps. The third nap, if taken, tends to be brief and in the late afternoon or early evening. But by six months of age, the vast majority of children (84 per cent) are taking only two naps; by nine months, almost all children are taking just two naps. No more third nap. On their first birthday, 82 per cent of children are still taking two naps, but by fifteen months, only 44 per cent are taking two naps. By twenty-one months, almost all children are down to just a single nap. See chapter 5 for more details about the emergence and disappearance of naps.

My studies also show that some babies are born to be short nappers and some are inherently long nappers. There is a strong genetic component to the control of naps in babies. Parents can interfere with a child's long naps by messing up the child's schedule, but they cannot make a short napper into a long napper. Here is the range: at six months of age, about 18 per cent of babies have total daytime sleep of less than two and a half hours, while 67 per cent nap between two and a half and four hours and 15 per cent nap more than four hours each day. If your first child was a long napper and one or both twins are short nappers, don't think you are doing something wrong!

> **If one of your twins is taking short naps, you might find that his bedtime hour has to be earlier than for the twin who is taking long naps. The solution is to synchronise your twins' sleeping schedules as much as possible. See chapter 3 and take a close look at the 'Institute Synchronised Schedules' on page 50.**

Not napping means lost sleep. Over an extended period of time, children do not sleep longer at night when their naps are brief. Of course, once in a while – when relatives visit or when a painful ear infection keeps the child awake – a child will make up lost daytime sleep with longer night sleep. But day in and day out, you should not expect to satisfy your child's need to sleep by cutting corners on naps and then trying to compensate by putting your child to sleep for the night at an earlier hour. What you wind up with is a bad-tempered or demanding child in the late afternoon or early evening. Your child pays a price for nap deprivation, and so do you.

SLEEP CONSOLIDATION

The third key component of your twins' healthy sleep is that it be 'consolidated', meaning that they get uninterrupted sleep that is continuous and not disrupted by awakenings. When awakenings or complete arousals break our slumber, we call it disrupted or fragmented sleep. Naps can become fragmented when we rely on 'motion' sleep in a baby swing or car or allow catnaps in a pram.

Ten hours of consolidated sleep is not the same as ten hours of fragmented sleep. Doctors, firefighters and parents, whose sleep is interrupted frequently, know this very well. Consolidated sleep is more restorative and therefore better-quality sleep.

The effects of sleep fragmentation are similar to the effects of reduced total sleep: daytime sleepiness increases, and performance measurably decreases. Among healthy adults, even one night of sleep fragmentation produces decreases in mental flexibility and sustained attention, as well as impairment of mood. The same is true for children.

But some arousals from sleep are normal. During partial arousals we stay in a light sleep and do not awaken; our child might make some sounds during such a period. During more complete arousals, adults might become aware that they are looking at the clock, rolling over or scratching a leg, but even in children, this awareness is dim and brief and they return to sleep promptly. Sleep interruptions also come in the form of protective arousals. For instance, when we have difficulty breathing during sleep, which can be caused by large tonsils or adenoids obstructing the air passage, we wake up. However, frequent complete arousals or awakenings are usually harmful because they destroy sleep continuity.

When children have frequent arousals, we call the problem 'night waking'. Often these are normally occurring arousals and the real problem is not the arousal but rather the child's inability or difficulty returning to sleep unassisted. That's where sleep training comes in. When we help our children learn the skills to get back to sleep without our parental intervention, these night wake-ups will be brief.

My research shows that at five months of age, the personality trait of persistence or a long attention span is the trait most strongly associated with the duration of daytime sleep. That is, parents describe their children as persisting longer in trying to do something or focusing their attention longer if they have longer naps. And at three years, children who nap longer are more adaptable; they can adjust more easily to changes in their environment, which is thought to be especially important for success in school.

SLEEP SCHEDULES AND TIMING OF SLEEP

Healthy sleep also hinges on the timing of sleep and the development of a predictable, consistent sleep schedule.

To better understand the importance of maintaining sleep

schedules, let's look at how four distinctive biological rhythms develop. The first rhythm is a wake/sleep cycle. Immediately after birth, babies are wakeful, then fall asleep, awaken and fall asleep a second time over a ten-hour period. These periods of wakefulness are predictable and not due to hunger, although what causes them is unknown. Thus a partial sleep/wake pattern or rhythm emerges immediately after birth. Sleep/wake patterns continue to change as the brain matures.

The second biological rhythm has to do with body temperature. In all humans, body temperature typically rises during the day and drops to lower levels at night. At six weeks of age, temperature at bedtime is significantly higher than later at night. After six weeks of age, as temperatures fall more with sleep, the sleep periods at night get longer. By twelve to sixteen weeks, all babies show consistent temperature rhythms. It is at six weeks of age when evening fussiness or crying begins to decrease from peak levels and night sleep becomes organised, and it is at twelve to sixteen weeks when day sleep patterns become established.

A third pattern is added by three to six months of age, when the hormone cortisol shows a similar characteristic rhythm, with peak concentrations in the early morning and lowest levels around midnight. Cortisol levels fall during naps.

Melatonin rhythmicity is a fourth pattern to consider. Initially, a newborn has high levels of circulating melatonin, which is secreted by the mother's pineal gland and crosses the placenta. Within about one week, the melatonin that came from the mother has disappeared. At about six weeks of age, melatonin begins to reappear as the baby's own pineal gland matures. But the levels are extremely low until twelve to sixteen weeks of age. Then melatonin begins to surge at night, and the hormone appears to be associated with evolving sleep/wake rhythms by about six months of age. (Melatonin supplements should not be given to babies or young children to make them sleep better; there is no evidence that they are safe.)

What's important to take away from this is that even at only a few months of age, internal rhythms are already well developed: sleep/wake pattern, body temperature, and cortisol and melatonin levels. In adults, a long night's sleep is most dependent on going to sleep at or just after the peak of the temperature cycle. Bedtimes occurring near the lower portion of the temperature cycle result in shorter sleep durations.

Sleep that occurs in sync with other internal rhythms is better-quality sleep.

Shift workers cannot sleep in sync with their naturally occurring biological rhythms, and the resulting poor-quality sleep can cause headaches and stomach aches. Jet lag is another example of sleeping out of sync with other biological rhythms in which your ability to focus and perform certain tasks is measurably decreased.

When thinking about sleep schedules in babies and toddlers, consider sleep to be 'food' for the brain, just as breast milk or formula is food for the body. You don't breastfeed on the run while doing errands; instead, you find a reasonably quiet space. The same should be the case for naps. You don't withhold feeding because it is socially inconvenient; you anticipate when your child might become hungry, and you try to have food ready at that time. The same should hold true for naps. You don't try to force-feed your baby when she's not hungry; you know a hungry period will naturally come. Same for naps. A parent coming home late from work would not make his baby wait until he arrived and could feed the child; he'd likely arrange to have someone else feed the baby! The same rules should apply for the bedtime hour; don't 'sleep-starve' your baby's brain by keeping her up too late.

I often tell parents to become sensitive to their child's personal sleep signals. This means that you should capture that magic moment when the child is tired and ready to sleep and falls asleep easily. The magic moment is shown by a slight quieting, a lull in being busy, a slight staring ahead and a hint of calmness. If you catch this wave of tiredness and put the child to sleep then, there will be no crying. I like the analogy of surfing, because timing is so important there, too – you have to catch the wave after it rises enough to be recognisable but before it crashes. But if you allow a child to stay up too late and crash into an overtired state, it will be harder for him to fall asleep and stay asleep because he develops a second wind. Also, it will be harder for him to fall asleep and stay asleep because he is trying to fall asleep out of sync with other biological rhythms. His ride to sleep then will not be easy or pleasant. Timing is most important! Remember, not every sleep wave is the same, and not every child learns quickly how to ride his sleep wave. But as with everything else, after practice, it occurs effortlessly.

SLEEP REGULARITY

The last key component of healthy sleep is for that sleep to come regularly. That is, once you have established a schedule for naps and bedtimes, stick to it! With twins, establishing synchronised sleep schedules and sticking to them with some regularity is essential, both for the twins and for you parents!

The best time for your twins to fall asleep at night is when they are just starting to become drowsy but before they become overtired. On page 39 you'll find a handy list of the things to watch for, the signals most babies give that they are ready to sleep. Of course, sometimes, due to long day care commutes or dual-career parents coming home late, it may be impossible to catch that magical drowsy state. The result is a bedtime that is usually a little too late.

Children will be better off if bedtime is at approximately the same time every night. It doesn't have to be exactly the same hour every night, but the range of time should be narrow: perhaps thirty minutes for young babies and sixty minutes for toddlers. More irregular sleep schedules are associated with more daytime sleepiness. It is thought that chronically variable sleep schedules might cause experiences similar to jet lag: nagging fatigue and cognitive disorientation. One study showed that children ages four and five with more variable sleep schedules were described by preschool teachers as not complying with the teacher's urging to join an activity, not showing enthusiasm for learning something, and arguing and fighting more than other children.

Don't beat yourself up if, unavoidably, your children occasionally go to sleep a little too late. But try to keep the bedtime fairly regular.

To extend the sleep-as-food metaphor, consider this: with these five key ingredients for healthy sleep in place, your twins will get the sleep nourishment they so desperately need to grow and to thrive. Now let's turn to the nuts and bolts of how to help them learn to get this sleep on their own!

PART II

Sleep Strategies for Twins and Multiples

CHAPTER 3

How to Sleep-Train Twins

The need for sleep is biological, but falling asleep is a learned skill. Sleep-training babies – singletons and multiples alike – is a system made up of five simple steps, which we'll discuss in this chapter. Fundamentally, this process is about sleep management: planning and organising when your children will sleep and helping your children develop the ability to fall asleep on their own. For parents of twins and multiples, this is especially important since helping your twins learn to soothe themselves and helping them get onto a schedule will ensure that you also get the rest you need.

Working together and getting other helpers (grandparents, babysitters, etc.) on board with your plan is essential. When someone breaks with the emerging routine or doesn't stick with the plan to sleep-train, you lose ground. Chapter 4 will detail the importance of teamwork – and ways to establish it.

> '*I just want someone to tell me what to do to get better sleeping habits because I want to teach them to my twins. I don't want to start too early but want to do it as soon as we can!*'

WHEN TO START SLEEP TRAINING

For the first few months of your twins' lives, you are likely and understandably going to be more concerned with their weight gain than with their sleep. In truth, feeding issues often push sleep issues off the radar with newborn multiples. This is the case with parents of singletons too, but more often than not, twins are born early and are often light for their gestational age. Babies born early are also more likely to have gastro-oesophageal reflux disease (GORD), so they might need frequent, small-volume feeds to prevent vomiting. Indeed, being vigilant about feeding twins every three hours is a good idea when you bring them home from the hospital; it is as if the periods of sleep are the unintentional by-products of the feeding schedule.

Still, even if it is not your primary focus early in your twins' lives, it's never too early to start sleep training, and the earlier you can begin to introduce the steps I outline below, the better. That said, for the first several months after you bring your twins home from the hospital, I urge you not to be *rigid* about sleep training; instead, you should be thinking of ways to *nurture* sleep in your twins and to encourage self-soothing skills. Self-soothing is the learned ability to fall asleep unassisted without protest or crying. And the earlier you start to teach it, the easier it is to learn it.

The five steps I detail below are aimed at twins under four months of age, so you'll see that we'll be dealing with sleep issues and sleep solutions as they appear and manifest in very young babies. Except for Step 2, which details the advantages of brief intervals of wakefulness, the steps are largely the same for older babies and children. You can start on the first day home from the hospital. But because biological rhythms, such as night sleep rhythms, emerge at or after six weeks and nap cycles emerge at about four months of age, you'll want to step up your vigilance and become more disciplined about instituting these steps between weeks 6 and 16.

SLEEP-TRAINING YOUR TWINS IN FIVE EASY STEPS

Step 1: Put the twins down to sleep drowsy but awake.

Twins who always fall asleep at the breast or on your chest become parent-soothed children who subsequently may have difficulty soothing themselves to sleep without your involvement at naptime and bedtimes and during normal arousals in the middle of the night. If they always fall asleep at the breast, on your chest, in your arms or in a swing, they are more likely to associate the process of falling asleep with those sensations and have difficulty falling asleep by themselves.

In contrast, when babies are put down to sleep drowsy but awake, they have the opportunity to learn how to soothe *themselves* to sleep, and throughout their young lives this will serve the whole family well.

Often, babies, especially premature ones, will fall asleep quickly during every feed. But when they are past their due date, if you always hold them until they are in a deep sleep, you deprive them of opportunities to learn self-soothing. The idea here is to shorten the duration of parental soothing so when they are put down to sleep they are drowsy but awake. Remember, if they are kept up too long, they will develop a second wind and get revved up instead of calmed down.

Sometimes you'll simply want to hold one of your twins as he or she falls asleep (doing so can be a wonderfully peaceful time for everyone and a rare chance to bond with one at a time), but as often as you can, try to put both your twins down drowsy but awake. If they cry hard, pick them up for soothing and try again a little later. If they make a quiet sound or whimper, do whatever your heart tells you: pick them up or watch and wait to see whether they fall asleep or begin to cry.

Raising twins is exhausting, so you will likely want to get help. Hiring sensitive, loving and caring people for child care is your goal. But adults with these desirable traits might have difficulty putting your twins down drowsy but awake. This is especially true for a person (a maternity nurse or a nanny) who sleeps in the same room with the twins. Be careful to see that they follow your guidelines.

Drowsy Signals

Dusk precedes night as drowsiness precedes sleep. An internal wave of sleepiness slowly rises. As the wave begins to develop, we might see drowsy signs or sleepy cues in our children, so watch closely. Watch for the development of the following drowsy signs to catch the sleepy wave as it develops:

- **Decreased activity:** Activity is a relative term when it comes to babies. When they get older, you'll be looking for less crawling or walking (and more sitting down mid-effort), but in young babies you're looking for less kicking and generally less squirming around.
- **Slower motions:** As with decreasing activity, be on the lookout for slow-motion movements and generally less energetic efforts.
- **Less vocalisation:** Crying is certainly one way babies can be vocal, but when crying increases, that may be a sign that you've let them stay up too long. The kinds of vocal signs that signal drowsiness come before the crying starts. Here, be on the lookout for less cooing and squeaking (whether in delight or in surprise).
- **Weaker or slower sucking:** If you are nursing or bottle-feeding your twins in an attempt to quiet them before sleep, you'll likely notice a less concerted effort on their part as they get drowsy.
- **Quietness and calmness:** Here I'm referring not only to a child's vocalisations but to the quiet that might come into his body as he gets drowsy. Quieting down and slowing down often go hand in hand.

- **Appearing uninterested in surroundings:** Babies are fascinated with faces. When your twins break from eye contact, that's a sure sign of increasing drowsiness. Likewise, when they begin to shorten their focus on whatever is interesting in their sight line, they are approaching the drowsy zone.
- **Less visual focus:** Along with a diminishing interest in their surroundings, drowsy babies' eyes will focus less (for shorter periods) on what has interested them and held their attention before.
- **Drooping eyelids:** This is a sure sign of drowsiness in babies and adults alike!

Signs That a Baby Is Entering the Overtired Zone

Fussing

Rubbing eyes

Irritability

Crankiness

Step 2: During the day, put twins down to sleep often, with only brief intervals of wakefulness.

At twelve to sixteen weeks of age, nap rhythms are developing and will eventually emerge around 9am and 1pm. But most babies under the age of about four months will want to and be ready to fall asleep more often and after a very short interval of wakefulness. Surprisingly, when they are very young, they might want to fall asleep after being up for less than one hour, and even when older they might want to fall asleep after only one to two hours of wakefulness.

Overtired babies and children become fussy or whiny or cry before they collapse into sleep because they feel the same discomfort that we feel when we are sleep-deprived: the smouldering headache, the feeling of being wound up tight, the dry eyes, the brain fog, the parched throat and the subtle muscle aches. But our overtired, sleep-deprived twins can't tell us what's bothering them. So to prevent the pain of being up too long and not getting enough sleep, keep the intervals of wakefulness brief.

As soon as you come home from the hospital with your full-term twins (or once they reach their due date, if they were born early) and through the first three or four months, your goal will be to experiment with brief intervals of wakefulness. Throughout the day, attempt to briefly soothe your twins and put them back to sleep (drowsy, but awake) shortly thereafter. Sometimes, because the preceding nap was very brief, you might decide to try this after only thirty minutes of wakefulness, but at other times the twins might have had a long nap and appear so alert that you wait until they've had more like ninety to one hundred and twenty minutes of wakefulness.

This is not an exact science, nor is it a by-the-clock nap schedule for young babies. On average, you'll be looking at a one-to-two-hour window of wakefulness, but this is only a guideline, not a rule. That said, it is also a ceiling, not a floor. No baby under four months can comfortably tolerate prolonged periods of wakefulness.

Brief intervals of wakefulness keep babies in a lower state of neurological arousal. In this state of being more relaxed, it is easier for them to learn self-soothing skills and they gradually become better able to fall asleep and stay asleep unassisted.

The better twins nap during the day, the better they will sleep at night. If they do not nap well, they develop a second wind of nervous energy that interferes with night sleep. Likewise, the better babies sleep at night, the better they will nap during the day. If they do not sleep well at night, they wake up in the morning too tired to take good quality naps. Remember, sleep begets sleep.

> **One to two hours of wakefulness for babies younger than four months of age is a guideline, not a rule. But it is also a ceiling, not a floor. More than two hours of wakefulness will overtire most babies of this age, and the result will be babies who won't be able to get to sleep and stay asleep easily.**

Initially, even if only one twin baby is drowsy, it makes sense to put them both down at about the same time. Later, especially for fraternal twins, you might have to make some adjustments to how you nap them because of individual differences, but for now, the rule should be: one down, both down.

Sometimes your timing will be off; you put them down to sleep too late or too early. It will take time for you to gain some experience. But practice improves performance, and if you are patient and stick with it, then you will see success with fewer though longer naps.

Sleeping Arrangements

When the twins come home from the hospital, I think that it's natural to place them in the same crib. After all, they have been together consistently in utero and will likely continue to enjoy each other's company. Remember, because their sleep rhythms haven't yet developed at this age, you probably will not see much difference between their sleep patterns. If you prefer to separate them when they come home from the hospital and place them in different cribs, I don't think that this will cause any problem.

Sometimes, several days after the expected due date, one twin might fuss or cry more and sleep much less than the other. To allow the calmer twin extra sleep, it might be a good idea to separate them so each has his or her own crib. More commonly, after several weeks or a few months of age counting from the expected due date, it is usually a good idea to move them into separate cribs because they are bigger and each twin needs more room.

Eighty per cent of the parents I surveyed put their twins in the same crib when they came home from the hospital for both naps and night sleep. After about four months, many of them separated their twins. Only about 20 per cent kept their twins in the same crib for more than four months.

In the beginning, one down, both down!

Sometimes one twin's colic or GORD will necessitate sibling separation to spare the sleeping twin; many parents separate their twins at naptime as a way to ensure that they don't disturb each other during these small windows of sleep opportunity but then bed them together at night as a way to help them both get used to periods of arousal and help them both learn to soothe themselves to sleep. I think this is a wise choice because if your twins' sleep has been protected and nurtured during naps, they will be better rested, calmer and more often able to find healthy sleep at night.

There are, of course, other considerations besides one crib or two. The Foundation for the Study of Infant Deaths (FSID) recommends that the safest place for a baby to sleep during the first six months is in a cot in a room with you. However, many parents believe in separate rooms for their twins (if they have room in their home for this), and others believe in the 'family bed', at least for the first several months of their babies' lives. These logistical concerns are really about parental proximity, and you will have to decide how comfortable you are with being apart from your newborn twins when they are so young. The middle ground is also a common choice: twins together in one room and at least one parent sleeping/camping out in their room at night in order to be closer for feeds and soothing. Some of you will make this choice to save your partner the disturbance of your getting up and down to feed at night. Others of you will find that you yourself can't seem to sleep without being able to quickly lift an eyelid at every noise the babies make. Again, these decisions are deeply personal and even culturally determined. Your parents and friends will no doubt share their opinions with you, but I urge you to do what you feel comfortable with. You will also want to be flexible. You have the right to change your mind or your sleeping arrangement as your twins' needs change.

If you decide to try a 'family bed', you will likely hear that your choice is controversial. Indeed, the American Academy of Pediatrics and the Foundation for the Study of Infant Deaths (FSID) discourages the family bed for reasons of safety, and you should discuss this subject with your health visitor or GP.

In my survey of parents of twins, only a few consistently used a family bed. But on a temporary basis, when one twin was ill or needed extra comforting to sleep better, the family bed might be used to help a twin get extra sleep. When combined with a cosleeper (a crib or mattress that can be attached to the side of the adult bed or in some way delineate protected space for the baby or babies on the adult mattress) and attention to the potential hazards of sleeping with your child, the family bed might give everyone a break and restore some calm in the family.

Step 3: Practise sleep routines.

Think of a sleep routine as a way to soothe your baby into a calm, quiet, drowsy state. Some parents always feed, burp, sing and rock their babies before naps and then give their babies a bath before bed; others do some or all of these things before trying to put them down for both naps and the night. *What* you do for a routine before putting your children down for a nap or for the night is frankly less important than *when* you do it, though the key here is to be consistent in your timing and the specific routine you use. Ideally, your soothing routines (not including a bath) should take from ten to twenty minutes; if you've been watching for signs of drowsiness to trigger your soothing routine, longer routines might well keep your babies up a bit too long or you might find they fall asleep in mid routine (which goes against the drowsy but awake rule!) Practise soothing routines as soon as you come home from the hospital so your twins learn to associate your routines with feeling drowsy and falling asleep.

Here are a few basic strategies that have a calming effect, either individually or in combination.

- **Rhythmic motions:** If you find sleep irresistible on a plane or train or in the passenger seat of a car, you'll understand how gentle, rhythmic motions can induce sleep in babies. Try rocking, swinging, gentle jiggling or bouncing one baby at a time. Or load both twins into car seats or a pram and drive/push them around the neighbourhood. But caution: don't let the babies fall asleep this way! Transfer them from your swing, sling, pram or the car before they nod off.

- **Gentle pressure:** There's nothing like feeling cosy and safe to make a baby (or even an adult) sleepy. Try swaddling or hugging your babies close to give them this feeling (cloth slings work well for this) for a short period before putting them to sleep. Baby massage – wherein you stroke and gently offer skin-to-skin contact (your hands to their bodies) – can also help before sleep time.

- **Sucking:** Most parents already know that a surefire way to relax babies – and therefore induce drowsiness – is to allow them to suck at the breast or bottle or to encourage them to use a dummy or suck their own wrist or finger(s). A dummy is, of course, a matter of personal preference. One problem that often arises with the use of dummies is that they fall out of babies' mouths easily, and before the twins are old enough to find the dropped dummy themselves, you'll have to be the one to help out. To this point, if your twins are ardent suckers, thumb or finger sucking is something to hope for: once they learn that their fingers and thumbs are right there at the ends of their hands, they can find them and use them without your help! Unfortunately, I don't know of any ways to encourage thumb or finger sucking other than swaddling your twins but leaving their arms free. I think some kids are just born to do this.

- **Sounds:** Babies love singing (lullabies or melodies), shushing ('shh' sounds), humming or quiet talking before falling asleep. Having heard their mother's voice in utero, it's often the case that Mum's voice – reading a book, telling a silly story or just chatting – can have a soothing, sleep-inducing effect on babies. Likewise, white noise – from a hair dryer, a vacuum cleaner, a fan or a noise machine – can help quiet babies down and bring on that drowsy wave.

- **Warm bathing, warm receiving blanket:** The majority of parents who filled out my extensive twins questionnaire reported that bathing their twins was part of their evening soothing routine. Relaxing (while being held or supported) in warm water and then being transferred into a warm blanket sounds wonderful, doesn't it? Many much older children still find this the most soothing way to end the day. Of course, there's no rule against bathing your twins before a nap, but bathing babies is an involved and longer process than most parents want to take on in the middle of the morning or day.

> *What* you do for a sleep routine is not as important as *when* you do it.

Consistent soothing sleep routines – even allowing for Mum and Dad's different styles of executing the same techniques – serve as a transition from light to dark and from active to inactive. There is not one routine that works best for all babies.

One father asked me whether it was always necessary to do everything in the routine that they had established; in particular he sometimes wanted to skip his twins' baths. I responded that he should do whatever he wanted. He agreed: 'I see the bath as a tool in the belt to use as needed.' The thing to remember and appreciate here is simple: if you initiate your routine when you notice that your twins are drowsy, you will help them associate their sleep routine with the biological sensation of drowsiness.

> 'The sleep routine that works best for us is . . . putting the boys down with a dummy, a much-washed cloth nappy next to their faces, and a thin cotton knit blanket over their bodies in a darkened room with a fan blowing. That combination

> *of things equals sleep to them, whether it is a nap or overnight sleep. They almost always instantly relax and get drowsy when they have all the elements in place.'*

Protecting Routines and Shutting Out Distractions
Newborns are sleepy for a few days after they are born (premature infants will remain consistently sleepy for longer). Because they are so sleepy, they appear to be very portable. For a few days or a few weeks, you can take them anywhere at any time and they will sleep through loud noises and bright lights. Nothing seems to disturb them.

But after a few days or weeks of age, counting from their due date, all babies become more alert and awake. They become more curious about and aware of their surroundings. They are more easily startled by the flash of a camera or a thunderclap. If they are in a situation where there is a lot of stimulation (people talking loudly, traffic noise, kids squealing on a playground, loud city noises, being jostled in a pram, or bright sunshine or city lights), they might have difficulty falling asleep easily and might not sleep well with all the noise. If the duration of this excess stimulation is too long, the babies stay awake too long and get overtired. Once overtired, they have trouble falling asleep and staying asleep.

In your attempts to establish sleep routines and frequent naps when they are very young, remember that it is the *duration* of wakefulness that interferes with your twins getting the sleep they need. Protect their newly forming routines and avoid sustained stimulation or distractions.

Step 4: Institute synchronised schedules.

Though I urge you to treat your twins as individuals and to work with them separately to meet their respective needs, one of the essential steps to sleep-training more than one baby at a time – and regardless if they are fraternal or identical twins – will be to synchronise their eating and sleeping schedules as early as possible. There is simply not enough of *you* to go around if you don't: you can't sustain your own health and sanity if you don't do yourself the favour of streamlining the sleep-training process with this important step. Parents of twins in my survey consistently stressed the importance of this part of the process. Though identical twins are often very much in sync with each other from birth, fraternal twins might present more of a challenge.

> '*Sleep schedules were so key to my sanity! I went from feeling the world was collapsing around me to feeling I could breathe again when the twins started to have a schedule!*'

Eating Schedules

Most parents of twins approach this sleep-training step in the following informal order: they start with synchronising eating schedules, then work on night sleep schedules, and then iron out the naps. This is not only a reasonable way to approach the process, it is often necessary. Most twins are born early, and your main concern in the early days will be to get their weight up. Many parents find that until their twins are at their due date, waking them every three hours to feed is the best and most successful strategy. If your babies are full term or close to thirty-seven weeks and are not particularly lightweight at birth, consider longer intervals between feeds at night, but you still might be feeding every three hours during the day. Discuss this possibility with your health visitor or GP because there may be other factors, such as gastro-oesophageal reflux disease, that require a frequent feeding schedule. Your twins might thrive with less frequent feeds if they can take larger volumes at each feed. If you are unsure about whether your twins are getting enough nutrition, frequent weight checks with your GP will give you the confidence to feed them less often.

The most common strategy for instituting a feeding schedule is: feed one, feed both. That is, if you determine that it is time to feed one twin, also feed the other, even if it means waking him up to feed him. Either way, the goal is to synchronise feeds so both are fed at about the same time and, hopefully, you and the twins can get some sleep in between the feeds. Whether it's breast milk or formula, a 'dream feed' or an awake feed, it's a good idea initially to try to feed both twins at about the same time. 'Never wake a sleeping baby' to feed doesn't apply to twins. Remember, healthy sleep will encourage healthy appetites. When twins are running on less sleep for fuel, no amount of food can make them less cranky or uncomfortable.

The age-old and popular saying 'Never wake a sleeping baby' doesn't apply to twins. In order to

**get their eating and sleeping schedules synchro-
nised, there will be times when you simply have
to wake one to do so.**

Night and Nap Sleep Schedules

Sleep rhythms mature as the brain develops. Regular nighttime sleep rhythms will begin to emerge at about six weeks post-due date; regular naps (usually at around 9am and 1pm) begin to emerge at about twelve to sixteen weeks post-due date. This is as true for big babies as for small babies. So even if your twins have dramatically different birth weights, you should expect sleep patterns to emerge at about the same age. Many parents think that sleeping well at night occurs when their child reaches a certain weight. But gaining weight is only the by-product of the more important factor, the passage of time. So as early as six weeks will be an appropriate time to try to enforce sleeping schedules.

In practical terms, this means you should be deliberate in your thinking. Set specific goals for getting your twins to sleep at certain times during the day and at night. Some parents find that writing these hopes down – making a list – helps galvanise the effort and also ensures that everyone on your sleep-training team (spouses, grandparents, nannies, babysitters, helpful neighbours) will understand your expectations for your twins' sleep.

You should expect sleep patterns to emerge at about the same age in your twins even if they have dramatically different birth weights.

The corollary of the feeding rule of thumb 'Feed one, feed both' is 'One up, both up' when it comes to instituting synchronised sleep schedules. That said, and as with feeding, if there is only one parent or person 'on duty' at a given time, it will be physically impossible to get both babies up at once. Naturally, understandably, there will be a little elapsed time between when you pick one up and tend to his needs and when you pick the second one up. The point here is not so much to be precise as to be mindful of the overarching plan: getting the twins onto more or less the same sleeping schedule. It's not realistic to have *exactly* identical sleep schedules and sleep routines for both twins. In real life, illnesses or holidays disrupt schedules. Schedules are derailed; sleep patterns crash to a sudden halt. But twins who have been sleep-trained will get back on schedule more easily and quickly once the illness or disruption has passed.

Let me be clear: when I say 'One up, both up', I'm referring only to the initial wake-up in the morning and to nap wake-ups. If you have to wake one up, wake them both up at these times. If one wakes up on his own at a time acceptable to your schedule, wake the other shortly thereafter. But if one twin wakes when she's not expected to – let's say she has a cold the other has not caught and she is having a hard time with coughing in the middle of the night – you should not also wake the other. Instead, try to make up the less well rested twin's sleep the next day by letting her rhythm and needs set the standard for the day. Or, as many parents in my survey reported worked for them, allow this twin the leeway to sleep a little bit longer in the morning. In this way, you will be allowing the twin who had overnight sleep trouble to catch up just a bit on her sleep; you can then try to proceed with your regular sleep schedule over the course of the day.

Whether one twin is sick or not, you should be prepared to factor some leeway into the schedule that you design. You might always allow one twin to have a little extra snooze time in the morning or at naps and enjoy the one-on-one time with the twin who needs less sleep. I advise that thirty to forty-five minutes of leeway is fine, but much more than that and you run the risk of throwing off the overall schedule. Maybe one of your twins consistently requires more soothing before being put down drowsy but awake. That extra time can be part of the leeway you allow in the routine. You'll simply have to make compromises when one twin awakens and the other twin is asleep or when one twin needs much longer naps or much longer time to soothe himself to sleep than the other. Remember, regardless of whether you are rigid or flexible according to clock time, your goal should still be to work with your twins' cues and drowsy signs.

To get a clear idea of how much sleep children of various ages need (and ways to synchronise what may be pronounced differences in your individual twins' needs), see chapter 5. Use these cumulative daily totals as a guide when you are trying to determine whether to let one or both of your twins sleep a little longer.

Most parents of twins advise that if there's one time to be rigid in trying to synchronise sleep schedules, it is the morning nap. They observe that if they are successful at synchronising the morning nap, the rest of the day's sleep schedule will go more smoothly.

As your twins get older, you might have to abandon your attempt to maintain a strict sleep schedule with or without leeway and instead adopt a more flexible or approximate sleep schedule if that works best for your family and your family's needs. For instance, if your twins have an older sibling who has to be at school or picked up at a certain time, Mum and Dad might decide to forgo the twins' rigid sleep schedule in favour of harmony for all the siblings.

Compromise between what *you* want and what the twins need is also a big factor in your ability to sustain strict synchronised schedules. When your twins need to nap but you are desperate for some fresh air or social contact with other adults, you'll need to weigh your priorities. Caregivers need care, too! Recharging your batteries – through time to yourself, a lunch date with a friend, exercise or whatever works for you – will ultimately help you to better care for the twins.

Think of it this way: creating synchronised sleep schedules can be limiting for you because they may force you to stay home at prescribed times, but they can also be liberating because once you can count on those naps or sleep times, you can make plans of your own for that 'free time'. Some parents use that time to sleep! Others arrange for sitters when they know their twins will be asleep and get out of the house to do something together or for themselves. Most of the parents I surveyed accepted imposed sleep schedules for their twins because they said they knew 'that it is for the twins' benefit and it will not last for ever'. But this knowledge does not make it any easier for you if you feel imprisoned in your home during naps and painfully miss your own social activities. This sacrifice of personal freedom may be hard. But the payoff in the present and the future is huge. Again, twins who have been sleep-trained early and properly will establish good sleep hygiene and habits and may be better able to be flexible and adaptable to their families' needs!

> *'We lived in New York City when they were babies, and while it was easy to get out and about, because I had the twins and because I wanted them to sleep, we rarely left the apartment for the first three months. This had a big impact on our adjustment to parenthood and family life. We realised sleep was crucial to all our happiness, but it did require some sacrifice in what we did and how we lived. Now my kids are great sleepers (generally), so the hard work early on definitely paid off.'*

Step 5: Make bedtimes easy; no more tears.

On paper, the appeal of sleep training looks attractive. In practice, however, some families cannot commit to it fully because they cannot establish schedules without a lot of crying. And for them, crying is unacceptable.

It's true that when you are trying to establish synchronised sleep schedules, one or both of your twins might cry or fuss at the designated sleep times. Maybe one is too tired or not tired enough, or maybe one just wants to play more with Mum and Dad. Inevitably, the question arises: is it all right to let one or both twins cry to see if they will settle down and fall asleep, and how will one child's tears impact the other's sleep?

In general, some crying by one baby twin, in the long run, will not disturb the sleeping of the other. From my surveys and research, it appears clear that the better-sleeping baby usually adapts quickly and ignores the crying of the other. For older twins, separation is sometimes needed at nap times because one twin cries so loudly and long. But when they are babies, crying for a few minutes at sleep times is fairly common and acceptable. It is also sometimes simply unavoidable, especially once they are about four months old.

Every parent has his or her own threshold for tolerance of crying, and personally I tried not to let my own children cry much in their first months of life. Listening to a baby (let alone more than one!) cry is very hard if you know that going to him and picking him up will soothe him. But crying – from both the baby's and Mum's perspectives – is not always hard. Sleeplessness is harder!

I offer you here three methods for dealing with crying that all promote self-soothing. Some parents of twins will modify them, combine them or use one method for one twin and another for the other. If you feel completely up-ended about the crying that can accompany putting your twins to sleep, have confidence that many parents of twins before you have found success with these methods. But note: none of these methods works well if you have missed the wave of drowsiness that should precede your twins' sleep. When they are overtired, children get wound up, and you might have more crying and less success with these methods. As always, first look for drowsy signals in your twins, and then experiment with these strategies and see what works for you.

Check and Console

Use this strategy any time after you have moved beyond feeding your twins every three hours. When you hear one of your twins cry, promptly attend to her by replacing her dummy, massaging, gently rocking the crib, reswaddling or shushing her, but try not to pick her up, talk to her or feed her. Because of your prompt response, your twin will not be really cranked up; you will be likely to calm her with minimal soothing. Because babies can sense and smell their mothers and might become more awake with the expectation that she will pick them up when near, I find that this method works faster and better when it is the father who does the checking and consoling. The goal is to allow the child some opportunity to return to sleep with minimal help from parents. After six months of age, your minimal soothing is likely to become more socially stimulating and counterproductive than when your babies are younger. Some babies start to sense that there is a game to be played: they cry, you show up!

Controlled Crying (Graduated Extinction)

Consider using this strategy at night after six weeks (from the due date) when you expect longer blocks of sleep at night and an earlier bedtime is emerging.

When your twin cries, wait for five minutes before going in to soothe him. Unlike checking and consoling, where you respond promptly, the delayed response with controlled crying or 'graduated extinction' means that your twin will likely become more upset. Therefore, with this method your soothing can and should take the form of whatever will calm your baby back down to a drowsy but awake state: pick him up, sing to him, breastfeed or rock him. The goal is to eventually soothe him to a drowsy but awake state, but if your baby falls asleep while you are soothing him, that's okay. Drowsy or asleep, you then put your baby down to sleep.

At that time or later, if there is more crying, you will wait for ten minutes before you return to soothe your twin. Repeat your soothing performance. And again put the baby back down to sleep.

At every subsequent time of crying, delay your response by an additional five minutes. There is nothing particularly magical about a five-minute interval, but some delay is necessary and consistency is key; you might want to try three-minute intervals. You might cap the maximum time of your delay to twenty to twenty-five minutes, or you might start out the next night with a ten-minute delay in your response time. Your expectation here is that eventually your baby will fall asleep during one of your delays. This begins the process of allowing your twins to learn how to return to sleep unassisted.

It is my experience that, again, this method works faster and better when it is the father who does the soothing. Even though feeding the babies is accepted in this method, if the father is the one to do the soothing, breastfeeding – which many babies prefer – is not an option. Some babies will settle down and get to sleep faster when the breast is not available to them.

The entire controlled crying or gradual extinction process may take a few nights or a few weeks. The process works faster when you start early in the evening, when drowsy signs first appear. Sometimes the repeated bouts of crying are overwhelming and you might decide that letting your twins 'cry it out' (see below) is the best option for speeding up the process of getting to 'no more tears'.

> *'For the first week, they often would cry for up to thirty to forty-five minutes. This would be through one five-, ten- and fifteen-minute cycle with consoling in between. By week two, they were usually asleep before the first ten-minute cycle had passed. By week three, they were down usually within the first five minutes. Now they go down within a minute or two. Sometimes they talk and play a bit longer, but they don't cry.'*

Crying It Out (Extinction)

The optimal time to use this strategy is after three to four months of age (post-due date). Perhaps this is when both parents must return to work full-time or with postcolicky infants (colic usually starts to dissipate at three to four months) or after parents see partial success with graduated extinction.

Extinction can successfully be used earlier, but most parents find it unacceptably harsh for younger babies. Extinction was used with some twins in my survey at five to six months of age after the due date, when the parents had suffered from becoming desperately sleep-deprived. At three to four months, many parents in my survey used extinction successfully.

Extinction means open-ended crying at night. The process is pretty straightforward: if you know that it is time to sleep and not time to feed, you ignore the crying, without a time limit. Initially, the baby will fall asleep after wearing herself out crying, but very quickly this process teaches the baby how to fall asleep unassisted *without* protest or crying. And the baby then stays asleep for a longer time.

A major fear here is that prolonged crying by one twin will disturb the sleeping of the other. Parents in my survey stated that the sleepy twin, surprisingly, almost always adapted to the crying after a few nights and slept through their sibling's protests.

Of course, another major fear is that you will harm your child by letting him cry. But as long as he is safely in his crib, letting him cry is only a means to an end of better sleeping. There is no published research showing that this procedure causes any harm to children. In contrast, there is no question that not sleeping well truly harms them.

If your twins' bedtime is early and naps are in place, the process of extinction usually takes three to five nights. In general, the parents in my survey describe the first night's crying to be thirty to forty-five minutes, the second night's ten to thirty minutes and the third night's zero to ten minutes. If their bedtime is too late or a twin is not napping well, the process may take much longer, or it may appear to work but the success is short-lived. Sometimes older children cry more on the second night than on the first, but the entire process still takes just a few days.

'We started around three or four months as fatigue from care and unpredictable sleep schedules reached the breaking point. The first night, our babies cried for about twenty minutes; the second for about ten minutes. They've slept through the night ever since.'

'My daughter cried for twenty minutes and then woke up at 4am and cried on and off for an hour and a half. The next night she went right to sleep and slept through the night and has ever since. My son cried for twenty-five minutes and then slept throughout the night and went down the next night without a peep. He has slept through the night ever since. I never thought it could work and work so fast.'

'At five months, we began [crying it out], and it only took three nights. They have since slept about twelve hours a night. This was a very difficult time for me and I cried hysterically, but it was worth it. The first night was the worst, and then it got better. They were sleeping through within a few days.'

Some families in my survey modified this sleep strategy by putting a top limit on the amount of crying they would tolerate. This is what I call 'modified extinction'. If you set a top limit, you might have peace of mind knowing that you are not committing to ignoring crying for ever. This helps the parents tough it out, and it often works very well for a sleep-disrupted twin. If you decide to use modified extinction, be careful to not set a top limit that is too brief. When you don't give your twin or twins enough time to really cry it out, you run the risk of training them to cry to that limit because a baby might learn that if he persists, he will be rewarded with more attention from Mum or Dad. In my survey of parents who tried this method, and in my experience, I think forty-five minutes is about the right minimum top limit.

As with controlled crying, many parents of twins find that they can train one twin using extinction even when the twins share a room. Again, the sleepier and more rested twin will sleep despite the racket! But when some families do extinction for only one twin, they separate them for a few days until the formerly bad sleeper is sleeping better. They then reunite the twins in the same room.

'In our experience, extinction works amazingly well with twins. We sleep-trained our twins in the same room (no need to separate them for sleep training) – they learned to go to sleep despite the other baby's crying. Our twins woke each other up for one or two days, but thereafter, they both fell asleep within one to two minutes and slept the entire night. I think twins need to be sleep-trained in the same room so they learn to be in each other's presence. If parents sleep-train the twins in separate rooms, the twins will

undoubtedly lose ground when they are placed in the same room again because they will still have to learn to sleep together.

'We utilised extinction for night sleep and graduated extinction for day sleep until the twins learned to sleep.

'Night 1: Both cried for forty-five minutes, and then they both fell asleep and slept the entire night.

'Night 2: Both cried for thirty minutes, and then they both fell asleep and slept the entire night.

'Night 3: Both cried for approximately ten minutes, and then they both fell asleep and slept the entire night.

'Night 4: Both cried for one to two minutes apiece, and then they both fell asleep and slept the entire night.'

As with the previous two methods, I have observed that there is less overall crying with extinction if, at bedtime, Mum leaves the house for a while and lets Dad listen to the crying. Why is it easier for the twins and the father? I think that the twins know – again, perhaps by smell – that Mum has gone and there is only Dad to soothe them. They are sleepy anyway, so they cry less. And of course, they know that Dad can't nurse them.

One mother of twins whom I talked to said she felt it was 'cruel to be kind'. She described how kindly going to her twins repeatedly at night to comfort them maintained a night-waking habit and ultimately was cruel to them because it caused them to have fragmented night sleep leading to sleep deprivation.

You should feel free to use more than one sleep method or a hybrid of your own making. There might be one night sleep method for one twin and another for the other twin. Or maybe use one method at bedtime but another method in the middle of the night or at naps. A common pattern for parents is to start with check and console, then try graduated extinction and then try extinction. But as I mention above, your tolerance for crying and your own subsequent sleep deprivation will be different from another's. There are many paths to our goal of a well-rested family.

CHAPTER 4

Creating a Sleep-Training Team

All new parents of twins need to get a little help, a little time off from their newly exhausting double duty. Getting help caring for your young twins is a key component of your successful adjustment to the new family dynamics. Anticipating the need for help and arranging it before you are desperate for it (even before the babies arrive) will also help you make better decisions. Remember that when you get severely sleep-deprived you will be less able to think straight, and that will impact the success of your sleep training. This point needs to be emphasised: prevention of sleep problems requires some clarity as to who will do what and when. Treatment of sleep problems requires strong willpower in addition to good organisation and planning. If you are already sleep-deprived when reading this book, have your partner read the book, help create a sleep-training plan and, of course, help implement it. Otherwise you, sleep-deprived reader, will have difficulty getting off first base.

Whether you get a maternity nurse for help in the early weeks or a nanny for the long term or simply take relatives and friends up on their offers to lend a hand with babysitting, you'll find that giving yourselves some time alone together (and alone separately) every now and then will rejuvenate you so that you can be at your best with your children and with each other. You've worked hard to have these babies – especially Mum, who has had to carry and deliver them! – so cut yourselves some slack and let others help you. Sleep training takes patience, and patience can be in short supply if your own needs are not being met.

That said, no amount of time away from the primary care of your twins will accelerate your ability to sleep-train them if you aren't yourselves in charge of the process, and if you aren't yourselves in agreement about how and when you want to try to do it. Indeed, you should consider yourselves the *core* sleep-training team, and those who are helping out need to take their cues from you. Whether you are reading this book before your twins are born or in between feeds or during naps once they are home from the hospital, it would be best for the whole family if you *both* read it. As the core team, you both need to be invested in the process and in agreement about your plans for sleep training.

'Try to be on the same page. Have discussions before the children arrive about your expectations and your goals. We talked about how we wanted to deal with breastfeeding,

> *eating issues, bathing, helping to maintain schedules, house-work and cooking, and even though we had to adjust and reconsider some decisions as time went on, being able to talk about these things was really helpful.'*
>
> *'It is hard to know which comes first, marital harmony leading to better sleeping or better sleeping leading to mari-tal harmony.'*

A BICYCLE BUILT FOR TWO

Many years ago, my wife, Linda, and I decided to get a tandem bike. We thought it would be fun to cruise around on it together, instead of riding some distance apart on our own bikes. We found one tandem that was sleek and fast – it had thin tyres, two drop handlebars, thin, aerodynamic seats and toe clips. It was something special to look at, but once we tried it out, we discovered it wasn't terribly practical for our needs. Crouched down behind the front rider, the person in the rear seat could see only the other's backside. We also both realised that we felt trapped in the toe clips. Explaining the design problems to the shop assistant, we considered a model he thought would be much more appropriate: the new bike had fat tyres and a drop handlebar for the front rider but an upright handlebar in the back; it had soft, wide, padded seats and clipless pedals. Functionally, this new bike was much better for our needs and our sizes. Picking it out together – and testing different models – was what led us to this 'right fit'.

Of course, the purchase was one thing, but now we needed to learn to ride it. We decided that I would ride in front – in tandemspeak, this role is called the 'captain' – and would therefore make the decisions about when to slow down, when to turn and when to pedal harder. Linda preferred to ride behind me in the role called the 'stocker', the person who largely concentrates on pedalling to supply the bike with power. Communication – regardless of who plays which role – is essential. If I did not clearly announce my intention to brake or turn, Linda might lose her balance or fall off. Linda also had to be able to make herself understood when calling for rests or for us to coast. Our helmets made it hard to hear each other clearly all the time, so we tried to devise a system of nudges and taps to signal different intents. Still, for this undertaking to be really enjoyable, we needed to be able to talk, not shout!

Happily, we discovered a battery-powered headset connection, and we could suddenly not only hear each other but swap observations and jokes and make plans for stops and rest as a team. With our headsets on and our roles defined, we practised and got better. We started to really enjoy the ride.

And so it goes with sleep-training twins. To extend the tandem bike metaphor: parents must work together to avoid potholes and make the climb to the top of hills. Together, you can then enjoy the ride down.

Twin Talk

Constant, clear communication is essential so that you'll be in agreement about what you're trying to achieve and how you'll try to achieve it. If you're not on the 'same page', one parent might keep the twins up too long when he or she is in charge. Or if you haven't talked about and agreed on what method you want to use to deal with the twins crying at bedtime, one of you might rush to check and console when the other thought that you were going to try graduated extinction. Chaos – and frustration – ensue! The straightest line to sleep-training your twins is to work together towards the same goal. Your ability to be consistent and coordinated – in the messages you are sending to your twins through your responses to them – is perhaps the biggest factor in helping them learn to soothe themselves and fall asleep without your constant help.

WHO'S IN CHARGE?

Having defined roles – understanding them and agreeing on them – is a big part of being a successful sleep-training team. Because she has carried, delivered and may be nursing the twins, I find that mothers are the best leaders or 'captains' of this effort, especially in the early months. If Dad has had to return to work after just a week or two off, Mum will also be the one who spends the most daily time with them and the one who will more quickly develop a sense of the twins' drowsy signals and an instinct for their respective sleep needs.

But when it comes to calling the shots about what your twins need, don't take the definition of 'captain' and 'stocker' too literally. The best teamwork is collaborative: fathers can and should be actively involved in the decision making and in the care of the twins. Fathers can sing lullabies, rock and swaddle the babies, offer bottles and give massages. Dads can do everything that mums can do, except breasfeed. Your family will benefit greatly if Dad is actively involved in the care of the twins from the very start. The captain's role is not to tell the stocker what to do but rather to be the person who is aware of the big picture of your twins' sleep and sleep needs on a daily basis. Likewise, the stocker should not simply be the passive helper but needs to take responsibility for and control of as much of the process as is workable in your particular family. There are as many ways to manage your shifts, your time and your respective needs as there are couples. If your work schedules allow, swapping tasks to allow each of you more of your own sleep can be beneficial for both your health and your marital harmony! Since babies can no doubt sense stress in the person holding and soothing them – and may become stressed themselves as a result – it makes sense to try to reduce your own tension through shift work and the sharing of responsibilities. Indeed, many parents in my survey reported that the more in sync they were, the more successful their sleep-training efforts. Some families devise a schedule for task rotation; others are far less formal about it. Some agree to split tasks instead of switching them.

Especially as the twins' biological sleep rhythms start to emerge at six weeks, fathers and mothers can and should try to share the burden of nighttime soothing. No parent can continually be the one to have badly interrupted night sleep! Plus, when Dad gets a chance to care for the twins on his own, he will quickly develop the soothing and care skills that he'll need to give Mum regular breaks from her sometimes daunting routine. Continuing to communicate will ensure that you are following the same course of action and working towards the same sleep-training goal.

> 'My husband and I work as a team planning family outings, picnics, holiday gatherings, weekends, day trips and many other things in our life: we simply do everything, 99 per cent of the time, around our kids' sleep schedule. When we make exceptions to this rule, we are well aware of the consequences – two cranky, overtired kids who would need to catch up on their rest at some point. It's not an easy lifestyle, and we know many couples with kids who think we are strange. It's better now that our twins are down to one nap, but it's still a constant choice: to be late for a picnic so our kids can have a long, restful nap; to rush home in the early afternoon on a Saturday so they can sleep in their cribs rather than in the car; to finish their first birthday party by 7:30pm, so they can go to bed; and so on.'

DADS AT BEDTIME

In addition to the marital harmony that can come from active and interested collaboration and communication, the parents who responded to my survey reported that sleep training went more smoothly and was established more quickly when fathers took on a very specific role: putting the twins to sleep at night from the very beginning. Some mums attributed this to the fact that their twins' fathers were less distressed by hearing the twins cry and were therefore more able to stick to an agreed-upon time for letting the twins 'cry it out'. Some couples said that dads were better at the 'tough love' approach. Others described Dad's bedtime routine as more effective because he wasn't responsible for the other daily twin care; he had more energy to draw on and to devote to this one daily – and important – task.

If a dad is home during the day, the same can be true of the nap time routine: Dad might have better success getting the twins to fall asleep on their own for the same reasons as above. But because sleep consolidation is so important to healthy sleep, it's important to get the twins to sleep early (before they get too wound up) and to help them have as much uninterrupted sleep as possible overnight. Naps the next day will come easier when the twins have had a healthy overnight rest. Use Dad's skill when it's most needed!

Whatever couples attributed this success to, they were definitely in agreement about one thing: if fathers or others are never involved in soothing the twins to sleep, the babies always associate falling asleep with being at Mum's breast or in her arms. This tight link between mother's feeding and soothing and falling asleep appears to make it harder for the twins to learn self-soothing skills, which become especially important when Mum is simply too tired to do it all herself.

> **Fathers are often more successful in getting their babies to sleep at night when Mum leaves the house for just a short while during the initial bedtime routine. Many think that this is because the twins can't smell or sense Mum and the soothing breast milk she might otherwise provide.**

If you decide to have someone other than Mum – and preferably Dad – responsible for bedtime soothing routines, try to start right from the beginning, even during the very early days or weeks, when your twins might still be very sleepy and no trouble at all to put down drowsy but awake. This might be as simple as passing each baby to Dad after nursing so he can do some soothing and put one down before Mum hands off the other twin. Or, if you are bottle-feeding your twins, Dad can give the nighttime bottle, soothe each baby and then put them down in turn. If the father does *not* develop the habit of helping out with the soothing – minimal though it may be – during these early weeks, then later, when the babies become more wakeful, Dad won't be as skilled and confident at the task and – my study shows – might be inclined to cede this responsibility back to Mum.

Your partner may not want to get involved with sleep training because he is dubious about the benefits, but when fathers actually see how much better their twins behave when they sleep better, they become believers:

'He admitted that in the beginning, he thought I was a little obsessed with the whole "sleep thing", but then he realised after seeing the effects of good and bad sleep – seeing that the girls were miserable when overtired and very happy and engaged when they were well rested – he quickly became a believer!!'

'Initially my husband didn't buy in to the rigid scheduling and early bedtimes; however, over time he saw that while it seemed counterintuitive it really did work.'

'It was definitely hard for their father when they used to go to bed by 7pm – he had only just got home within the hour. But I was persistent and explained to him that I would bear the consequences the next day. Also, he could see on the weekends that it made a huge difference in how much fun they were to play with when they were tired versus rested.'

But Mum needs help – she needs Dad (or someone else) to take this task off her already overfull plate! So get Dad on board right away. I recommend that fathers step up to the plate and begin soothing their twins at bedtime as soon as the twins come home from the hospital. Forget washing the car. Forget changing the oil. Fill up the family's emotional and physical tank with sleep to get the machine going!

Some mothers in my survey said that they actively did not want their husbands involved in the daily care and sleep training of their twins because they had had to work so hard to have their babies in the first place, and they felt it was 'ungrateful to complain' or to ask for more help (a sentiment that seemed to coexist with delaying the process of sleep training as well!). These were most often women who had undergone extensive assisted reproductive technology (ART) to conceive their twins, so it is understandable that they felt so grateful for being mothers in the first place, but if a mother too rigidly takes on the role of the leader or the caller of shots, she may innocently (or deliberately) make a barrier that keeps the father limited to a helper role, if he has any role at all. This is not a sustainable arrangement! In the long run, this exclusion might invite a lot of marital discord, and it sets Mum up for being the primary caregiver of the twins at all times.

'Our months and months of ultrasounds, pills, charting and hard work had finally come to fruition. I, for sure, was more hesitant to sleep-train my babies, whom I had tried for so long to have!'

THE RIGHT KIND OF HELP

Some parents choose – if finances allow – to hire a maternity nurse for their twins' first few weeks. Others have a relative come to stay to help out in those early days and agree to let that person take the overnight 'shift' until Mum has recovered from delivery. Getting this kind of early help can be extremely positive as your new family adjusts to your very different and very new routines. But it's often the case that this person – the maternity nurse, the grandmother – will think of her role as trying to keep the house quiet overnight so that the new parents can rest. With that as her goal, and especially if she is sleeping in the same room as the twins, she might rush to soothe the twins as soon as they make even a peep, and if your arrangement is that she will bring the twins to you for overnight feeds, she will bring them to you more often than necessary. She might also rush to quiet one twin in an effort to protect the sleep of the other, and that impulse is also understandable.

Though there's no harm in this for the first few days home from the hospital (newborn mewling *is* irresistible!), keep in mind that as your twins become less sleepy and their biological sleep rhythms start to emerge and mature, the rush to soothe and/or feed them to keep them quiet will not help the sleep-training cause. It's also important to understand that most parents report that one twin's fussing does not usually upset or disrupt the sleep of the other. Remember, they have been cohabitating for quite some time and are used to the other's movements. When your well-meaning helper rushes in to keep things quiet, the twins will be learning that help and soothing arrive when they fuss. Once the maternity nurse or grandparent leaves you on your own, you will be left dealing with the twins' expectations!

A happy compromise in these situations is to explain to your maternity nurse or your helpful relative that you want them to respond only to the twins' outright crying and you want their peeps and squeaks and snuffling around to be monitored but not always attended to. If you explain your expectations for how often each twin will want or need to feed, you can also request that your helper not bring the babies to you until the agreed-upon amount of time between feed has elapsed. It's hard to be strict about these things – and many parents have told me that even with the best of intentions they give in to the noise they can hear in the next room and get up to help the helper! – but if you keep in mind the goal of trying to help the twins soothe *themselves*, you'll hold the line more often.

Of course, if you are not getting overnight help but are yourself sleeping in the twins' room to be on call for their overnight needs, try to follow the same advice: resist soothing and attending to every small noise. You'll absolutely want to respond to clear crying or your twins' discomfort, but learning to differentiate natural nighttime noises – which sometimes even include short cries – from noises that require your intervention will serve you well now and into the future.

The same rules apply during the day: you'll need to explain to anyone who offers to help you out that keeping your adorable twins awake past their expected nap times will actu-ally make things harder for you once they leave. Teach your helpers to recognise drowsy signals and explain your routines for putting each twin down for naps drowsy but awake.

Explaining these things – and enforcing them – can be especially fraught when the twins' grandparents are the ones helping you out. Most grandparents 'can't help themselves' when it comes to picking up, soothing and playing with their new grandchildren. If your repeated requests to protect your twins' sleep go unheeded, you might decide that the kind of help the grandparents provide isn't the kind you need right now. Later, when sleep patterns have been established and you've helped your twins learn to get the sleep they need (see chapter 5 for average sleep times for children of different ages), you can welcome their help again!

> **Most parents of twins find that one twin's restlessness or interrupted sleep does not markedly disturb the other's sleep, even when they are in the same crib. Especially when they are very young (under four months), both fraternal and identical twins tend to be undisturbed – or disturbed only briefly – by their sibling's fussing. As twins get older and bigger, putting them in separate cribs may be necessary to give them the physical room they need – to kick, to roll around – as they sleep, but even when they are in the same crib, don't rush to soothe one twin for fear that his cries will automatically wake the other. Experiment with their tolerance for the other's noise: you might be surprised at what your twins can sleep through!**

THE SLEEP LOG: A KEY TEAMWORK TOOL

I've never known parents of newborns – singletons or multiples – to be *absolutely* consistent about sleep training right from the start. The truth is that some parents swing back and forth between firmness and permissiveness often, and they cannot make even their best intentions stick for any period of time. Don't beat yourself up if this describes you. It's natural to want to be there for your twins, and you may have worries – about colic, GORD or prematurity – that will make it harder for you to resist stepping in to soothe one or both of them. Of course, there will also be situations, such as when one or both twins are sick, when frequent soothing will be necessary. In these cases, don't worry that you're derailing your sleep-training efforts. You can pick up the trail again when the twins are feeling better.

Very often, however, it is not your willpower that is the problem but rather your own sleep deprivation that clouds your perspective. You might confuse your twins' sleep patterns: just as you can forget which twin you breastfed first at the last feed, you can easily forget which one slept longer at the last nap and even which one prefers rocking and which one needs swaddling. Or wishful thinking – that they are sleeping better than they really are – muddles your thinking about each child's actual behaviour.

Many parents of twins use feeding charts to help them keep track of how often and how well each twin is nursing or eating. Some charts can be downloaded from the internet to help you do this. The corollary for keeping track of sleep is a simple chart called a sleep log. A sleep log can be an important tool in helping you document what you are *really* doing and how your child is *really* responding.

Creating and maintaining sleep logs for your twins is easy; all you need is two notebooks of plain or graphed paper. The logs should be made up of a series of bar graphs showing on each day when your child was awake, asleep, quiet in the crib (or bed, down the line) and crying in the crib. On the horizontal axis, show the day of the week and on the vertical axis, the time of day. A more detailed written diary can often make it hard to see the forest for the trees, but with a sleep log each bar represents a twenty-four-hour snapshot of a day, and the graphic view of all the bars allows you to quickly and clearly see trends in sleeping patterns for each twin.

I recommend keeping your twins' sleep logs in the rooms where they sleep (perhaps taped individually over their cribs if they are sleeping separately), so that the logs are always on hand when you are thinking about recording the sleep your twins have just had or the time in their cribs awake (or crying) as you go in to get them up. Have your helpers – your babysitters, your nanny, your relatives and neighbours – fill out the sleep log for each twin when they are taking care of them. This will help them stay on task – in tune with your instructions – and help you see what went on while you were gone. As patterns emerge, you can adjust bedtimes or nap times to keep up with your twins' individual sleep needs.

'I [used a sleep log] mostly to provide consistency between my husband, babysitter and mother.'

'The chart was one of the best ideas we came across. It kept everyone on the same page without wasting time with explanations. One glance at the daily chart, and anyone could see what was going on that day (i.e. status quo or one missed a nap and should go down for bed early).'

'The sleep log was extremely helpful. It was helpful for two reasons – (1) it forced us to pay attention to sleep cues from the babies. (2) It helped us to create a schedule that worked for both babies. We would keep one baby up a little later in order for both of them to sleep at the same time.'

'It was very useful to see the pattern that was developing in the eating/sleeping cycles. It helped us to be able to predict and then stick with a routine.'

'It helped to map improvement (or otherwise!) and therefore to keep optimism up.'

Here is an example of a sleep log. As you can see, this baby is starting to have clearly decipherable blocks of sleep, with quiet time – and less crying – before and after each period of rest.

SLEEP LOG EXAMPLE

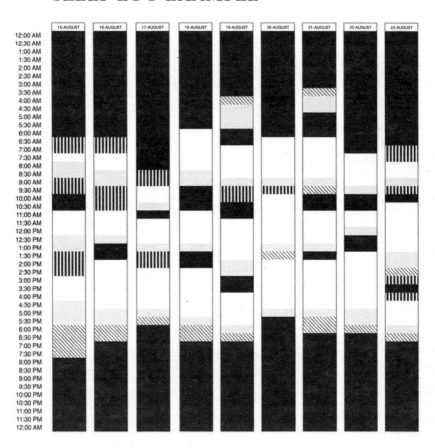

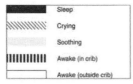

Sleep

Crying

Soothing

Awake (in crib)

Awake (outside crib)

TEAMWORK WINS

There can be little doubt that the challenges of rearing twins will add stress to both your days and your marriage. When you factor in the possibility of prematurity, colic or GORD, baby blues or postpartum depression, an older sibling who requires your attention, relatives who interfere and weather that prevents your strolling outdoors, it's a wonder that anyone ever survives the parenting of twins! The universal key to managing well and keeping your sanity and sense of humour will be teamwork. Teamwork, more than anything else, will also go a long way to preventing and correcting sleep problems.

CHAPTER 5

Children's Sleep Needs at Different Ages

N o sooner have you mastered catching drowsy signals in your twins and come to rely on seeing them at certain times of day, than their sleep needs and rhythms will change and you may find you need to adjust your expectations and routines. But knowledge is power, so having a general sense of when your twins' needs will change and what you can expect in terms of sleep at various ages will help you anticipate the changes and prepare or react accordingly.

The following table shows, on average, how long children sleep at different ages. These are sleep totals. Within each subsequent section of this chapter, we will look more closely at how these totals tend to break down at the same ages in terms of nighttime sleep versus naps.

Most of the data for this table were gathered in my study of more than two thousand young children in the Chicago area in 1980, but the results from other, earlier studies from England, California, Japan and Minnesota are much the same. It seems clear that despite cultural and social changes and such modern inventions as television, DVDs and computers that shape our contemporary lifestyles, the age-specific durations of sleep are firmly and universally rooted in our children's developing biology.

How Long Should My Twins Sleep?

AGE	TOTAL SLEEP HOURS
Birth–weeks 1–2	15–17
Month 1	13.5
Month 2	14.5
Month 3	14.5
Month 4	14.5
Month 6	14
Month 9	14
1 year	14
2 years	13.5
3 years	12.5
4 years	12
5 years	11

Of course, some children will require more sleep and some will need less, so it is always more important to look at each of your twins' mood and behaviour, especially at the end of the day, than to expect these numbers to be exact for your individual children. Use these sleep totals as loose guidelines as you observe sleep in your twins and try to help them get more of it. Consult the sections below for detailed information about each of these age groups.

NEWBORN TWINS
(Due Date to Week 2, Post-Due Date)

If your newborns are sleeping for close to a total of fifteen to seventeen hours within a twenty-four-hour period, they are probably getting the sleep they need, even if that sleep doesn't match up with when you'd like to get some sleep, too! Simply put: during the first few weeks of life, babies do not have – and therefore you will not be able to distinguish – any clear rhythm or pattern to their sleep. Actually, since many twins are born early, the only discernable pattern to be found in their sleep is that it comes in between feeds! Indeed, most health visitors will give parents of premature or even slightly early twins clear directives: feed them every three hours to get their weight up. As a result, feeding drives everything and periods of sleep will be just a couple of hours at a time until you can start to extend the time between feeds and thereby blocks of sleep as well.

Because of this lack of clear patterns – or because life feels like one giant march from one feed to the next – this is a time when most parents feel more than a little discombobulated. But these early weeks are also precious: the world will in many ways stop or at least recede from focus around you. Many parents report that when they look back at the very early days and weeks of their twins' lives, they can remember very little aside from constant feeding, nappy changing, trying to catch some sleep themselves – and a magical mood and feeling within the family that come from shared, intense experience and shared awe at what you have created! As jarring as it may be to have these two new people in your lives and in your home, and as difficult as it can be to recover physically from their delivery, the first two weeks of new life can be surprisingly peaceful.

> For the first few weeks of your twins' lives, they will need approximately fifteen to seventeen hours of sleep in a twenty-four-hour cycle, which will likely come in between feeds.

Whether your twins are premature or full term, whether they are fraternal or identical, what is universally true is that it takes time for sleep rhythms to develop and sleep needs to express themselves. Until babies are close to six weeks post–due date, nighttime sleep and naps will have little definition and demarcation. So, in the beginning, you might not see any differences in sleep patterns between fraternal twins, even though they might be genetically programmed to show different sleep rhythms when they get older. Indeed, your fraternal twins might have similar sleep rhythms at this early point, but they might not. Identical twins usually have more similar sleep rhythms, and they will tend to stay this way as they get older.

> The internal sleep/wake clock that regulates when we feel drowsy for night sleep and naps develops in a predictable fashion independent of

whether a baby is born early or on its due date. This development is about brain maturity, not about weight, so even if your twins are of dramatically different weights, their sleep rhythms will emerge at about the same time.

The sleep/wake internal clock develops automatically, but it does not guarantee quality sleep. Quality sleep requires nurturing by parents. And as we've discussed earlier, it is never too early to be on the lookout for drowsy signals and to be sensitive to your twins' sleep needs right from the start.

Most newborns are sleepy all the time – they sleep often, and they can sleep seemingly anywhere and through all kinds of noise and distraction – for several days after birth; premature babies will likely remain sleepy until at least their due dates. Shortly before or after their due date, your twins will become more alert and wakeful. They will have more wide-eyed looks and regard your face with more intensity. They will show more curiosity and sensitivity. In either case, just because they *can* nod off anywhere and anytime does not mean that you should let that be the norm. Your twins will sleep better right from the start if the room is dark and quiet.

SYNCHRONISING FROM THE START

As you learned in chapter 3, successful sleep training of twins depends greatly on synchronising their sleep schedules. At this early date – when schedules are determined largely by feeds and not by sleep – let the feeding schedules be the trigger for synchronisation. If you feed both twins at about the same time, you will be allowing them sleep at about the same time as well. To do this, you might sometimes have to wake a sleeping twin to feed her. Other times you may allow one twin to snooze a little longer while you feed his sibling, because he needs more sleep. Allowing for perhaps twenty to thirty minutes of leeway, your goal right from the beginning should be to have them on a fairly synchronised feeding schedule so you do not spend all your time feeding your twins. Feed one, feed both. One down, both down.

NEWBORN'S CRYING

In the first few weeks of life, your twins' alertness and wakefulness will increase. With this increased awareness, however, can come moments of unexplained fussing, irritability or crying. Premature babies are more likely to have gastro-oesophageal reflux disease (GORD), so you should talk to your GP about whether medication should be given. For most newborns, the crying might appear to be related to hunger because sucking at the breast or bottle often calms the baby. However, we know that sucking is soothing and sometimes it is the sucking itself (for example, on a dummy), not the breast milk or formula, that calms the babies. These bouts might appear to be due to abdominal pain because the twins might draw up their legs or pass more wind. Babies tend to swallow air when they fuss, though, so the wind they pass might be the consequence of the fussiness, not the cause. These crying jags or bouts of fussiness are perplexing and also sometimes distressing (especially when everyone is operating on less sleep than they are used to), but unless they are protracted and your baby is completely inconsolable, they are very normal (see page 94 for more information about colic).

Loud and insistent cries should always be attended to because a twin might be in distress, hungry, thirsty, wet, soiled, cold or too warm. Whether during sleep or while your twins are trying to fall asleep, quiet calls, whimpers, short, spontaneous cries and other sounds that do not seem to be demanding should probably be ignored. Try not to jump at every peep. Many parents of twins (or maternity nurses or helpful grandparents) respond too promptly out of the misguided fear that these quiet sounds will always escalate and disturb the quieter twin. This is especially common when you (or another adult) are sleeping in the same room as the twins. Sometimes a prompt response to quiet sounds is necessary, but usually, if left alone, the noisy one will calm down, or, even if he gets a little worked up, the quieter one will learn to sleep through his twin's disruption. Remember, these two have been sharing space for many months and some jostling and disruption are the norm for them both. In these early days and weeks, noise from a sibling (or movement, if they are sharing a crib) is different from new and prolonged environmental noise and distractions.

When the twins are a few weeks past their due date, the problem with responding too promptly to every sound a twin makes during sleep is that you run the risk of interfering with that twin's ability to learn how to soothe himself back to sleep unassisted. Additionally, the twin might learn that if he calls out more at night, he gets more attention from Mum or Dad or the maternity nurse. As discussed in chapter 4, if you hear your twins at night and are unsure how to proceed (and if it is definitely not time to feed them), I think it is better for the father to check out the situation than the mother. The more the father is involved, the faster the twins will learn self-soothing. If you are unsure whether they really are hungry or not, give a bottle of expressed breast milk or formula and see how many ounces they consume and how quickly they take it. This should give you clues to tell you whether or not they really were thirsty or hungry or simply wanted company!

If one twin is extremely loud or regularly cries for a long time, some parents separate them during sleep periods, but many observe that if they wait it out, the quieter twin adapts and learns to sleep through the sounds of her noisy neighbour.

FOUR TO EIGHT WEEKS OLD
(Post-Due Date)

As your twins get older and more awake and alert, you'll begin to notice several changes in their sleep habits. The total number of hours they are likely to want and need to sleep will first drop to about thirteen and a half hours and then increase to fourteen hours. At about six weeks of age (from their due date), your twins' biological sleep rhythms begin to express themselves; the beginning of a distinguish-able and organised night sleep rhythm starts to appear. Of the needed thirteen and a half to fourteen hours, perhaps eight or nine of them will be during the night (though not consecutive yet) and five to five and a half will be naps dur-ing the day. Most parents of twins put their twins in separate cots at this point to allow each twin needed space to move and stretch without kicking or disrupting the other.

As discussed above, before six weeks of age, the longest single sleep period is going to be perhaps only two to three hours, and that block might occur any time during a twenty-four-hour period. At six weeks, the longest single sleep period may well lengthen to a miraculous four to six hours. Most often, this longer stretch of sleep occurs at night or during evening hours, usually starting before midnight. In the early weeks of their twins' lives, many parents wonder if this moment will ever come. But it will! Night sleep organisation happens automatically and is independent of your method of feeding your twins or other parenting practices. One twin might settle down at night before the other. Be patient; soon both will sleep longer at night. You should still expect multiple night feeds (or crying that necessitates checking on them), so you won't yet be getting uninterrupted night sleep yourself, but at least you can enjoy four-to-six-hour blocks of uninterrupted sleep or quiet time in the evening.

When your twins are about six weeks old (from their due date), they will begin to settle into a more recognisable sleep pattern and sleep training in earnest can begin. Of the thirteen and a half hours that they may be sleeping at this point, five and a half of those hours will likely be during the day (many short naps) and the balance of eight hours will occur at night (though not uninterrupted yet!).

CRYING AND COLIC

In addition to being more awake for longer periods and asleep for longer periods, from four to eight weeks of age (from their due date), your twins' irritability, fussiness and tendency to easily cry peak. These behaviours can occur anytime, but usually they are worse in the evening and night hours, especially before midnight – just when you were hoping they'd start to sleep that longer block. Some babies are a little like this, and others are a lot. Those who show a lot of these behaviours are said to have colic or extreme fussiness. If one of your twins is extremely fussy and the other is not, it may now be necessary to separate the twins at night. Though in the earlier weeks your twins seemed to be able to sleep through anything, loud and persistent crying may now really disrupt the sleep of the noncolicky twin.

Colic is defined as more than a total of three hours per day of irritability or fussiness requiring soothing to prevent crying, or crying itself. These behaviours occur on more than three days per week and last for more than three weeks during the first three to four months in a healthy baby.

> **In my study with families of twins, almost 30 per cent reported that at least one of their twins was extremely fussy or colicky. It is rarer (9 per cent) for both twins to have colic.**

In some of my earliest research, I discovered that babies with colic have more difficulty falling and staying asleep. Trying to put them down drowsy but awake may not work until their colic has been resolved. But this does not mean you should not try to be aware of drowsy signals or emerging sleep rhythms in your twin who does not have colic.

If one or both of your twins have colic or are extremely fussy, you can't tend to their needs simultaneously! Necessarily, you will learn to tolerate a little mild fussing or crying from the twin without colic. This twin may soon learn to soothe himself to sleep or sleep through his sibling's crying simply because you can't be in two places at once! Of course, if both of your babies have colic, teamwork will be all that much more essential. You can't care for two distressed babies on your own. Ask for help. Get help. Accept help. And then use the time your helpers give you to do something for yourself.

'Allow yourself some downtime. When Dad gets home, make a run to the shops or go for a short walk. Even if it's just ten to fifteen minutes, that helps restore your sanity.'

'I think it largely depends on the mother, but for me, having help in the first few months was critical to my sanity. The other thing I strongly suggest, but had trouble doing, is trying to spend a little time alone. I had such a hard time giving up control to someone else. Still, spending time alone, whether to read, get a pedicure, take a walk, etc., is a necessity. It isn't optional. It's critical to the mother's sanity. For me, doing something for myself every now and then makes me feel like a woman, not just a mother.'

'Try to get out of the house for a little bit without the kids, even if it's only for half an hour.'

'Any time you can give her a break without guilt, please do. I do have help from my husband and family in watching the girls, but I feel guilty about it. If my husband lets me sleep later one morning, I feel like I need to reciprocate. It would be nice to feel that there were no strings attached.'

Everything begins to improve after six weeks of age. After the six-week peak of alertness, wakefulness, irritability, fussing or crying passes, your twins will be more settled at night. And there's yet another reward for your patience: your babies will now start to make real smiles – they will smile in response to your smiles!

NINE TO TWELVE WEEKS (Post-Due Date)

Between two and three months, your babies' sleep needs and rhythms will shift yet again. During this developmental stage, they will likely need a little more overall sleep (fourteen and a half hours instead of thirteen and a half to fourteen hours as in the previous weeks), with more of the total hours of sleep occurring at night.

Your twins will now likely start to extend their nighttime sleep to a total of possibly nine to ten

hours (though usually not uninterrupted) and may sleep four and a half to five hours during the day. They may need an hour more sleep than they needed just a month ago. Night sleep is lengthening, but day sleep is shortening.

As early as several days or, more often, a few weeks after the six-week peak of wakefulness and fussiness, the internal sleep clock begins to shift nighttime drowsiness to an earlier hour. Your twins will now want to go to sleep earlier at night. Instead of falling asleep at 9, 10 or 11pm, they will want to fall asleep at 6, 7 or 8pm. It won't be the same time every night, but it will be an earlier time. Remember, this trend is controlled by the internal timing mechanism that regulates sleep rhythms in the brain. So watch your twins carefully earlier in the evening to see when they are getting a little drowsy: slower body movements, less sparkle in their eyes, less social animation or drooping eyelids. It's to be expected that there will be some mild differences in your twins' sleep times at night – especially with fraternal twins, whose individual biological sleep needs might now begin to show themselves – but if they are rubbing their eyes or acting fretful, recognise that they have become overtired and attempt to put them to sleep earlier the next night.

It's at this stage that I most often hear parents rationalising keeping their twins up 'a little longer' in the evening in an attempt to 'tire them out so that they'll sleep better'. In the proverbial trenches, this impulse is understandable: nine to twelve weeks into this process you are weary of the nighttime wake-ups and feeds and may well be desperate to have your twins sleep through most or all of the night so that you can sleep too! But it's crucial to resist this temptation and to re-member that healthy, uninterrupted sleep will come more easily and regularly to a baby who is not already overtired. It may seem counterintuitive to you, but it's proven: sleep begets sleep! Watch for drowsy signals, and try to catch the sleep wave. If your twins develop a second wind (their bio-logical response to exhaustion), you'll have more trouble get-ting them to sleep and getting them to stay asleep.

> **What's 'early' in terms of bedtime for your family may or not be early for another family. Don't worry about or monitor how other families are managing. Watch your own twins' mood, person-ality and behaviour and adjust their bedtimes and nap times accordingly.**

The stubborn fact is that there are long-term disadvantages if you always or often put your twins to sleep a little too late. They accumulate a sleep debt, which gets them cranked up and fussy near the end of the day, when they run low on sleep power. This explains the all-too-common lament: 'My babies were sleeping well until they got to be around two or three months. After that things began to fall apart.' Cumulative sleepiness over two to three months causes the sleep tank to go almost empty in the late afternoon or early evening. But of course, there is no sleep gauge for you to monitor like the fuel gauge on your car. Your eyes are your best defense: watch your twins for signs of drowsiness, and attempt earlier bedtimes. Here are two commonly utilised strategies for instituting earlier bedtimes:

1. **Make the bedtime a little earlier.** Choose a fifteen-to-twenty-minute-earlier bedtime and stick to that slightly earlier time for four to five nights. After four to five nights, incrementally move bedtime an additional fifteen to twenty minutes earlier. You may find that you need to adjust their bedtime only by that first fifteen- or twenty-minute increment, but most babies who are running low on sleep need more than that time to catch up on their 'fuel'. Repeat this process until you reach a bedtime where the twins go down calmly and fall asleep easily.

2. **Make the bedtime much earlier.** Choose a new, much earlier bedtime that might be *an hour or more earlier* than the twins (and you) are used to. The twins will show improvement because they are now sleeping more in phase with their biological circadian sleep rhythm. You might not want to keep this super-early bedtime too long, because it might backfire and cause the twins to consistently wake up too early in the morning. If so, regroup. By trial and error, find a sweet spot between the original too-late bedtime and the new too-early bedtime.

My observation is that parents who successfully utilise early bedtimes have more pleasant morning times with their babies and rarely experience major bedtime battles, frequent night wakings or other sleep problems. They also report that their marriage is stronger because they have more private time as a couple in the evening and at night. The babies benefit because they are raised by well-rested parents who are more able to cope with real-life challenges. But the price you pay for earlier bedtimes is spending less play time with your babies at night, and this can be disappointing for a parent or parents who come home from work too late to see their twins awake before nightfall. Because sleep is vital for healthy brain development in our babies, I do not think it is too high a price to pay. Preserve and protect their sleep in order to enjoy the rest of your time together.

> *'Although I was disappointed when the boys started going to bed at 6:30pm because my husband and I were going to be able to spend only one hour with them in the evening, I learned it was selfish to keep them up for our entertainment.'*

THIRTEEN TO SIXTEEN WEEKS (Post-Due Date)

Between three and four months of age, the overall amount of sleep your twins need won't change too much, though they will perhaps need and be able to get another half hour to hour of sleep at night and perhaps slightly less overall during daytime naps. But even if there is not much of a shift in overall sleep times, there is one important development you can expect at this time in their lives: your twins' internal timing mechanisms will develop a daytime sleep pattern, and discernable naps will now emerge! You'll see them moving from catching sleep in fits and starts during the day to having perhaps three defined naps.

THE MORNING NAP

Up until this point, your twins' naps have likely been brief and not very predictable. But now, as the intervals of wakefulness during the day are lengthening, a regular morning nap will appear. Initially, it might start around 8 or 8:30am. Later, as their bedtime becomes earlier and they wake up better rested from longer night sleep, the morning nap will begin around 9am. If you have not already done so, now is the time to try your best to have naps at home or in some other dark, quiet place. The twins' awareness of environmental stimulation and their curiosity are keen, and this will interfere more and more with good-quality naps.

Keep in mind that *when* your twins' nap occurs is probably more important than *how long* it lasts. Your goal is to start your soothing to sleep for naps when the nap sleep rhythm is starting to rise. Catch the wave by being in the right place at the right time. Initially, the morning nap may be regular but brief (forty to fifty minutes), and the rest of the naps unpredictable and also brief.

THE MIDDAY NAP

Shortly after a regular morning nap appears, a second, midday nap develops as the internal timing mechanism for sleep further develops. Initially, this second major nap might start around 11am or closer to noon. Later, after four to six months of age, as the morning nap lengthens, the second nap settles into a starting time slot of 12 to 2pm. By six months of age (post-due date), the morning nap and the midday nap are each about one to two hours. Some children – especially babies who were colicky in the earlier months – develop this second nap rhythm when they are a little older.

Some children who go to bed too late and wake up tired do not develop these predictable naps, or, if they are predictable, they are too short (much less than one hour). Some twins who go to bed early and whose parents have perfect timing still have brief naps until six to nine months of age because of the genetic control of nap duration. The point here is that there is a lot of variability in nap patterns, especially the second and third naps of the day.

Of course, there is also sometimes considerable variability between your two twins' individual nap needs. Parents of identical twins report less schedule variability because the twins share similar nap patterns naturally. Fraternal or identical, however, most parents initially try to synchronise naps strictly and place both children in the same room. Sometimes, of course, it becomes clear – especially to parents of some fraternal twins or if one has been colicky in her earlier months – that separation and/or leeway for nap schedules works best. Some parents, mindful that naps will not emerge at the same time but rather build on the one that has come before, are very strict about the first nap but more flexible about the second.

AND SOMETIMES . . . THE THIRD NAP

Many babies have a minor third nap around 2 to 4pm, depending on how the major morning and midday naps have gone. This third nap is often brief and more irregular in terms of when it occurs and whether or not it is needed. Because this third nap is variable, your twins' nighttime bedtime might also be variable. If they've taken a third nap, their bedtime will be a little later in the evening. Rigid adherence to the clock for bedtime is a common mistake because it ignores the variability inherent in daytime sleep. Think of your twins' bedtime as likely to occur within a range of times. Watch your twins' behaviour and personality between 4 and 5pm to determine whether they should go to bed at the earlier or later end of the range you have determined for the bedtime hour. Between three and four months of age, the bedtime range is often between 5:30 and 7:30pm, depending on how the twins look at 4 to 5pm (starting to get drowsy or not, cranky or good-humoured). How they look at 4 or 5pm is largely affected by how they napped during the day.

The thirteen-to-sixteen-week-old period is a time of some flux, so you should not be a slave to your twins' nap and night sleep schedules. You are trying to help establish patterns and synchronise your twins' sleep schedules, but do allow yourselves some fun! Being rigid about when and where your twins will sleep every single day will wear you out just as quickly and surely as sleep deprivation does. As a general guide, keeping your twins up past their nap or nighttime sleep time once or twice a month is not a problem. Once or twice a week is another story; that kind of too frequent disruption will wreak havoc on the routines and patterns you are trying to establish.

'I had a lot of help the first three months, and then it all went away abruptly. It was scary to do it all alone. With my older child I had established a nighttime routine with a bath, pyjamas, book, song, the whole lot. When my nurse was with me, we did the same with the twins, and my husband did, too.

'But when they were gone and I was alone, it just took too long with the two babies. I ended up throwing the long "wind down" out the window; I started bathing them in the am. Their sleep routine ended up consisting of a bottle and some soft music. I realised that kids don't need a long routine. They ended up going to sleep just the same.'

FOUR TO SIX MONTHS (Post-Due Date)

Between four and six months, your twins' overall sleep needs will remain in the fourteen-and-a-half-hour range, with perhaps yet more of that sleep coming (uninterrupted) in the night and less during the day than in earlier months.

But even though the overall need for sleep hasn't changed much, this age range will bring with it an exciting new development: at this stage of their young lives, your twins' daytime naps will get longer. Whereas up until now, they have had many naps of shorter duration, when they are between four and six months of age, their two major naps will stretch to one to two peaceful hours! At this stage, for some twins, it may be the morning nap that is the longest, but for others, it is the midday nap.

In terms of nighttime feeds, there is great variation at this developmental stage. You may find that your twins still need to be fed twice, once or not at all. Before you rush in to feed them in the middle of the night, however, consider the following: your twins' internal timing mechanism has developed to the point where they are cycling at night between deep sleep and light sleep. During some light sleep periods they may become partially awake, and they will sometimes make sounds during these partial arousals. If you constantly rush in to soothe or feed them, you might wind up with twins with night-waking habits. As the twins become more social, their attitude will shout, 'Thanks for coming to me; let's play!' As adorable as their smiles and invitations to play may be, understand that interrupted sleep for your twins due to frequent night awakenings is unhealthy sleep when compared to uninterrupted or consolidated sleep. Small bits of sleep are not as restorative as long blocks of sleep, even when the total duration of sleep is the same.

THE WITCHING HOUR

If they have been going to sleep too late, have been getting fragmented sleep from receiving too much attention at night or are not napping at home in dark, quiet rooms at the right times, your twins might show signs of being overtired. Overtired really means sleep-deprived. They will become a little crankier, irritable, rough around the edges, clingy and demanding, and have an easy tendency to fuss or cry. This is especially and most dramatically so near the end of the day, when they are running out of sleep energy. This is the witching hour: tired, wired and all fired up. Being more vigilant about putting your twins down when they are initially getting tired – both at naps and at night – will decrease your experience of the witching hour. As one parent told me, 'At about three and a half to four months, we started to get really confused because they would scream and fuss between 7 and 9pm. We then realised that their natural bedtime was 6:30. It changed our lives!'

If your twins are in day care and you come late to pick them up, you might miss seeing this cranky time. They might already have developed a second wind, and this burst of energy combined with their joy to see you might mask the signs of being overtired.

WHEN ONE PARENT PULLS DOUBLE DUTY

At some point in your twins' young lives, one or both of you will have to go back to work, and that work might get you home late in the evening, perhaps too late to be helpful during the bedtime routine. Many parents in my survey reported that becoming the sole bedtime routine parent was a little scary – and complicated, since physically getting both twins ready for bed and calmly off into slumber is difficult for only two arms to do! As with all things twin, flexibility – both with yourself and with your established routine – seems to be the key to making the transition from two parents to one at bedtime. You might find that your soothing routines will necessarily have to get shorter or start earlier, you might decide to bathe your twins in the morning (a wake-up routine!) instead of the evening or you might decide to hire help for this critical part of the day.

> *'I was afraid and nervous to start doing bedtime alone [when my husband went back to working late]. After only a few nights, I knew something had to change. I started a new routine – I would let the boys crawl up the stairs to their room, and we'd read two stories before lying in their cots awake. This was a very hard transition, mostly for me, I'm sure! The first few nights they would scream when I left the room. I would leave for five minutes, and if they were still crying, I would go back in and pat them on the back and say "goodnight". I would repeat this until they fell asleep, adding five minutes to each interval of wait time. The first night they cried for about an hour off and on, but after only a few nights, it took about fifteen minutes of crying. It seemed that after only two weeks, there was no crying at all. They began to recognise the routine – they would grab their blankies and say, "Night, night".'*

SIX TO NINE MONTHS (Post-Due Date)

By six to nine months, night and day sleep rhythms are well established, so it makes sense to ask the question, 'Am I letting my twins sleep as their biological rhythms dictate, or are we still out of sync?' That said, you have two children, and sometimes those two babies will have different rhythms, so do not expect perfection! The other question you can ask yourself – and one that is likely easier to answer – is, 'Are my twins getting enough sleep overall?' Research shows that the average total number of hours that six-to-nine-month-olds need to sleep is fourteen to fourteen and a half hours, but your twins may need more than that. Look at their mood and behaviour at 4 to 5pm. Is this the 'witching hour', when things tend to fall apart? If so, they need more sleep.

> **Six-to-nine-month-olds need a total of fourteen to fourteen and a half hours of sleep, and most parents find that approximately three to three and a half of those hours will occur during daytime naps. Most six-to-nine-month-olds take at least two daily naps, and you can expect that each nap will last as long as one to two hours.**

Around six months, your twins' naps should lengthen. As before, you should be more concerned with *when* naps occur than with how long they last, but you can expect that your twins' naps – usually the morning and second naps – will each last from one to two hours. The morning nap might get longer before the midday nap stretches in length.

Naps at this age can be tricky, and badly timed naps can have a negative snowball effect: too much sleep late in the day can throw off the bedtime routine, late-to-bed twins might not sleep as well or have consolidated overnight sleep, and the next day will start for everyone with some sleep debt! The good news is that you can tweak your twins' nap times over several days to get things back on track. That is, you can rig the snowball effect to work in your favour as well. For instance, if your twins' first major (morning) nap is present but occurs early, for example, between 7:30 and 8am, the second nap will also start early, probably well before noon. Babies on this schedule will likely need a third afternoon nap, which *might* disrupt or delay the hoped-for early bedtime. But when a reasonably early bedtime is in place, your twins will be able to comfortably tolerate longer periods of wakefulness in the morning and their morning nap will shift to a start time of about 9am. This later morning nap will allow the second nap to start closer to noon or 1pm – and then that third nap might not be needed. It might look or feel like a chicken-and-egg situation, but my research and experience show that earlier bedtimes are the cornerstone of quality for both overnight and daytime sleep.

'The biggest challenge we have had has been with daytime sleep. The girls have been very good at soothing to sleep initially but always seem to wake up about thirty minutes

into the nap. By dinnertime, they are always overtired and miserable. But we started putting them to bed much earlier over the last few weeks. As a result, the morning nap has started to become longer and more consistent.'

At this age, many parents will have a strict approach for the morning nap and a flexible approach to sleep scheduling for the second midday nap. Usually they put the twins down around the same time for that first nap but then allow leeway for the second nap. In this way, when one twin wakes up first, parents will pick him up and allow the other twin an additional twenty to forty minutes of sleep. If the second twin is still snoozing away after that extra time, most parents report that in the name of reasonably synchronised schedules, they wake that sleeping second baby. Especially with fraternal twins, who may have different biological sleep needs, allowing this kind of leeway will give the sleepier twin some needed extra sleep and grant him the quality rest he needs to be able to get to sleep later in the day or at night. Of course, this kind of leeway might also open up a precious window of alone time with the less sleepy twin – rare moments when you can affectionately interact with only one baby and not feel the burden of caring for two at the same time.

Sleep problems often emerge between six and nine months of age because babies develop more 'self-agency'. This means that they become more wilful, persistent or determined to do what they want to do. If they want to push a truck and you want to change a nappy, it's now harder to distract them. If they want to fight sleep in order to have more fun playing with you, they will try harder to force themselves into a wakeful state to enjoy your company. Even though they have more self-agency, you still have the ability – and the power – to encourage or discourage sleep. There is a direct connection between how you behave and how your twins behave. Not all play is alike: calm, soothing, slow-paced time together will encourage sleep; roughhousing and animated play are likely to do the opposite. Ask yourself: am I soothing them to sleep, or am I interfering with their sleep because they enjoy my company?

NINE TO TWELVE MONTHS (Post-Due Date)

As your twins approach their first birthday, close to eleven to eleven and a half of their needed fourteen to fourteen and a half hours of sleep should be had at night, and if you have been sleep-training them, this can certainly be uninterrupted sleep (for you, if not completely for them).

Your twins will also now likely be taking two major naps each day: one in the morning and one at midday, for a total of perhaps two and a half to three hours. At this stage, a third nap in the late afternoon will almost certainly interfere with a reasonably early bedtime. When they were younger and taking that third nap, you likely had a later bedtime, but now is the time to both get rid of the third nap and move bedtime a little earlier. Think of a range of bedtimes for nine-to-twelve-month-olds as between 5:30 and 7:30pm. Moving your twins' bedtime a little earlier – even by ten to twenty minutes – can make a huge difference. Failure to do so will cause a sleep debt to accumulate and the twins will gradually begin to show rough spots between 4 and 5pm, followed by bedtime battles, night wakings or early-morning awakenings.

A small number (about 20 per cent) of nine-to-twelve-month-olds might go from two naps to one nap. If bedtime is reasonably early, it is the morning nap that will start to disappear, and the midday or early afternoon nap will be long and restorative. If their bedtime is late, however, this change from two naps to one can be really problematic: because they have had a too-brief night sleep, they need a morning nap. But if the morning nap is the only one they take during the day, nobody will be happy in the late afternoon. If one or both of your twins are refusing a second daytime nap, make sure to put them to sleep earlier in the evening so that the one nap the next day can come later and last longer. To the extent that you can control it, try to keep babies under a year old to two naps – a morning and a midday or early afternoon nap.

Special Occasions

All this talk of sleep schedules and the need for naps of certain lengths can be taken too seriously. Get out of the house during the day with your family, and go ahead and keep the twins up late on special occasions! Trust in the fact that the better they sleep on routine days, the less disruptive the exceptional days will be. But these special occasions should probably occur once or twice a month, not once or twice a week. After these disruptions of sleep schedules, if they behave over-tired, a 'reset' back to the old schedules might require a super-early bedtime for one night only. See part III, 'Troubleshooting', for specific tips and ideas for resetting or adjusting schedules to deal with special occasions.

ONE TO TWO YEARS OLD

Unless your twins were extremely premature, the effects of prematurity have diminished considerably by now, so you might consider this age range, and subsequent age ranges, as their chronological age, not their corrected (post-due date) age.

One-year-olds need about fourteen hours of sleep in a twenty-four-hour cycle. Most parents of twins report that their one-year-olds get approximately eleven and a half of these needed hours at night and perhaps two and a half through naps. It is between the ages of one and two, however, that many children naturally reduce their number of naps from two (morning and midday) naps to one midday nap.

My research shows that on their first birthday, about 80 per cent of babies are taking two naps a day. By fifteen months, about 40 per cent of babies are taking two naps a day and by twenty-one months, only 10 per cent are taking two naps a day.

It is also at this age that differences in biological sleep needs between fraternal twins will be very apparent. Indeed, transitioning from two naps to one can be especially difficult with fraternal twins because they might make this transition at different ages. Even still, the overriding concern for most parents of twins is to maintain the same nap pattern for both twins. It just isn't practical to have one twin take one nap and the other twin take two naps.

For babies close to one year of age (twelve to fifteen months), you can help them make this transition together even as you continue to put them down for two daily naps (and even if you strongly suspect or know that one of them will not sleep well or long with a second nap). The trick – as with so many of the scenarios above – is to put them both to bed earlier at night. The twins will wake up better rested, and this will naturally shorten the morning nap. Gradually, that morning nap will disappear for both babies. Another solution is to go to a single morning nap and gradually push it to a later and later start time so eventually this single nap is occurring at midday.

If you are trying to help one sleepy twin transition to only one nap a day in order to synchronise his schedule with a less sleepy sibling who really already needs just one nap, the transition process might take as much as a month to take hold.

If your twins are closer to two years old (fifteen to twenty-one months), you might more abruptly try putting them both down for only one midday nap even though one twin was sleepy in the morning. Families who have the luxury of child care help or lots of help from family members can allow the children to have completely different nap schedules.

But when daily help is not in the cards, most families choose the single midday nap for both children, even though one twin would clearly prefer two naps. Parents of identical twins usually breeze through this transition because the genetic control of sleep/wake rhythms keeps them on the same or very similar sleep schedules.

As in earlier days, you can tell if your twins are getting enough sleep by how they appear and act around 4 to 5pm. If they look and act well rested at that 'witching hour', they are getting enough sleep. If they are routinely cranky or irritable during that time, they are simply not getting enough sleep and you will need to put them both to bed earlier to help them wake rested to face each new day.

> *'I get home between 6 and 7pm. After the babies were born I made an effort to get home earlier to make sure I could provide some relief support at the end of the day. Now that we have gone to a super-early bedtime (6pm), I usually miss them at night. This is unfortunate and upsets me sometimes, but I know it is only temporary and in the long run everyone is better off. On the flip side, I get to see them in the morning and everybody is well rested and I get to do the morning feed.'*

TWO TO THREE YEARS OLD

Two- and three-year-old children should still be taking a single nap at midday, lasting about one to two hours. The ideal bedtime is early enough that they appear well rested between 4 and 5pm. Their overall sleep needs will likely amount to twelve and a half to thirteen and a half hours.

One problem that emerges around this time is climbing out of the cot. With twins, it is not practical to return the climber to his cot over and over again because the protest crying and the repeated parental intervention are likely to disturb the sleeping twin, who might well be in the same room. If both twins are climbing out of their cots, it is nearly impossible for one parent to corral both of them back to their cots and remain cool.

Cot tents, which are used in America, are designed to keep a child in his or her cot. Some parents hate the idea of a cot tent because it reminds them of a zoo cage. But often it takes only a few nights for a child to adapt to the cot tent, and surprisingly, he or she often enjoys it and wants to help zip it closed. However, it still might be necessary to put the twins' cots in separate rooms so that the one in the cot tent does not overly disturb the other twin.

Another problem that emerges around this age is the sleep setbacks that come with dealing with illness. The twins are now surely more social and interacting more with other children. They are sharing more toys and germs. They will therefore get more colds! When they are sick, you'll want to give them all the attention you can, both during the day and at night. Common colds last three to ten days, but the acute phase usually lasts twenty-four to seventy-two hours. After the acute phase passes, their fever – if they had one – is lower and their discomfort is less, but they are still slightly sick and may well very much want your continued attention. But I always tell parents – of twins and singletons alike – that when the acute phase passes, it's back to boot camp for sleep, even though they might still have a little cough or drippy nose. Usually one 'reset' night with a super-early bedtime will do the trick and get them back into their previous good sleeping mode. If you give prolonged extra attention at night for a week or two for every little sniffle, they will get way off schedule and way overtired. This will make it hard for you to return them to the previous good sleeping patterns.

THREE TO FOUR YEARS OLD

Between their third and fourth birthdays, about 50 per cent of children stop napping and will want to get all of their needed twelve hours at night. In my study, on their fourth birthday, half of children were still taking naps, though not every day (about five times per week). If your twins still want to nap at this age, watch out for too many scheduled activities that might interfere with naps or interfere with reasonably early bedtimes. Dropping their one nap should be a natural thing instead of something forced because of their busy days!

Bad sleep habits can sneak up, especially during long sum-mer days. If the time required putting your children to sleep is too long (too many bedtime stories, requests to go to the toilet, or demands for curtain calls for more attention) or you are trying to make the transition from cots to beds and they do not want to stay in their beds, you might need to implement some sleep rules to encourage your twins to sleep when you know they will be tired and to sleep well. Every family's 'rules' will be different, but the key is to set up a few rules that your children can understand and remember. Some families make the rule that their children must stay in their beds, close their eyes and try to sleep until a certain time that the kids have been taught to recognise on the clock. Other families institute a rule that the kids can't leave their rooms until a certain time or until music comes on from a radio set to an appropriate hour.

You might make a colourful poster that lists your family sleep rules under a heading that uses your twin's names: 'John and Daniel's Sleep Rules'. Place the poster on the wall in their bedroom to serve as both a reminder to them of what is expected at night and a reminder to you to be consistent. Such a poster is more powerful than you can imagine. Recite your family sleep rules at nap and nighttime, and be clear with your children about what will happen when they cooperate and when they violate the sleep rules. For cooperation, they receive a reward or treat. Try this: put a large glass bowl filled with small sweet snacks on top of the refrigerator. In the morning and after a successful nap, they get to have one treat if they cooperate with the rules. You might also find that star charts work well too: a certain number of stars might equal a larger treat, a toy or a special event. In this way, both immediate and delayed gratification come from cooperation. For 'sleep rules' to work, you have to pick powerful motivators!

For no cooperation, some privilege should be restricted. I don't think that creative items and activities such as art, music, books or playtime should ever be restricted. But perhaps a favourite truck or doll will be put out of reach if the child does not cooperate.

PART III

Troubleshooting

CHAPTER 6

Breastfeeding Twins: Special Challenges, Special Tips

This chapter was written with Nancy Nelson, R.N., ICBLC. Nancy is a nurse and lactation consultant who has been with my paediatric practice for more than twelve years. If you take Nancy's advice, I am confident you can avoid the frustration and heartbreak described by some mothers and instead have great success breastfeeding your twins.

If you choose to breastfeed your twins, the responses to my surveys as well as our paediatric experience prove that breastfeeding them is not only possible but can be wonderful and enjoyable, too. That said, there are certain obvious – and some less obvious – challenges with breastfeeding more than one baby at a time (whether simultaneously or consecutively), and you may find the demands of the double duty to be daunting at first.

Premature babies – which twins often are – tend to have weaker sucking abilities and higher incidences of gastro-oesophageal reflux (GORD), both of which make for longer and more frequent feeding sessions. Caesarean delivery – a common delivery for twins – is associated with a delay in initiation of lactation, and that can obviously complicate your efforts to breastfeed your twins. The physical stress of feeding two babies around the clock (combined with your own lack of sleep) can really ratchet up your anxiety level. In turn, anxiety – and sleep deprivation – can diminish your breast milk supply!

I certainly do not want to give the impression that breastfeeding twins is always difficult, but it *is* important to understand why there might be difficulties ahead. The more you understand why breastfeeding twins can be more of a challenge than breastfeeding singletons, the more likely you will be able to get the help that you need. It's my hope that the information and tips in this chapter will help bring the tension down several notches and that you'll soon be able to focus on enjoying your new family more!

'In the early months, feeding your babies drives everything. It is the most time-consuming, exhausting and often frustrating part of caring for your babies. When they are premature, you are hyper-aware of how much they are eating, when they are eating, keeping them awake to eat, if they are possetting, are they gaining weight, etc. Successfully emptying a 45- or 60-ml (1.5- or 2-ounce) bottle is a victory, especially if they keep it all down! That said, I think it may be even more difficult for parents of multiples

to separate sleeping from eating . . . that is, they believe it's necessary for a baby to have a nice, full belly in order to sleep longer at night. I had to fight this logic myself time and again and remind myself of the science. I was always shocked when one of mine would be so tired in the evening that they would only take a few ounces of their bottle, and I would put them down convinced that they would wake up early for the next feed because of hunger. Quite the contrary, sometimes they slept longer! I finally had to use an adult comparison and think, "If I'm exhausted and go to bed without eating very much that evening, do I wake up at 1:00am needing a meal?" No! My body needs sleep and will eat later.'

PREMATURITY

One hurdle to successful breastfeeding is prematurity, which is a common occurrence with twins and multiples. Indeed, most multiples in my survey were born before thirty-seven weeks' gestation.

This hurdle may be low if the twins are only slightly premature (thirty-four to thirty-six weeks' gestation) or quite high if they are very premature (thirty-three weeks and younger). Although it's easy to forget, prematurity affects the mother as well as the twins. Mothers of premature twins in my survey reported feeling more tentative about getting out and about with their babies because they wanted to protect their children from the risk of infection and illness.

That's a good impulse, of course, but when it keeps mother and children away from most other human contact and indoors for days, weeks or months on end, it's not good for anyone!

> *'Since the twins were born seven weeks early they required round-the-clock nourishment for the first couple of months. Although they were healthy, the risk of medical problems was increased and we spent a lot of time indoors, isolated and sleep-deprived.'*

Even in those babies born close to term, a medical complication might mean that one or both twins will need to stay in the neonatal intensive care unit (NICU), and that can delay breastfeeding or make breastfeeding more difficult. As if feeding issues weren't enough of a challenge, worrying and dealing with complications from prematurity drive sleep-training concerns further off the radar.

> *'When our twins were born, we were committed to exclusively breastfeeding them. The first nine days, while they were in the NICU, this meant that I had to travel to them every three hours. After my initial three days in the hospital, I and my husband or other helper had to travel approximately fifteen minutes to the hospital. There I would spend twenty minutes apiece nursing each baby separately*

and another twenty minutes pumping while my husband provided the supplemental feeding. It took approximately ten minutes to wash the pumping and feeding equipment and to store any extra pumped milk. Then, assuming we did not have to speak to hospital staff, we would take fifteen minutes to get home. Now home, if we spent twenty minutes taking care of ourselves (eating, drinking, showering), we had eighty-five minutes left to get undressed, fall asleep, sleep, get dressed and repeat the cycle. Dealing with lactation consultants, meeting with the orthopaedist who was correcting Baby A's clubfeet, making a shopping list and making important decisions with my husband about if, when and how to supplement, all ate into those precious minutes of sleep. We were in complete survival mode, and that was before the girls were even home.'

'When you have been through so much fear and anxiety about delivering premature infants, it is hard to ever think you could care about sleep training.'

Depending on gestational age, one or both of the babies may not be ready to take any oral feeds initially and may instead require tube feeds (using your expressed milk or a special formula). With a hospital-grade breast pump, however, you can help your milk come in and help your supply stay up.

As the babies get closer to their due date, their ability to coordinate sucking, swallowing and breathing improves, and one or both may progress to oral feeds in the hospital. Hospital staff will want to closely monitor your twins' nutrition intake and might recommend or require some bottle-feeding to be done in addition to breastfeeding. A common protocol involves feeding at the breast for ten minutes, pumping for ten minutes and then giving the baby a bottle with pumped breast milk. As your premature twins improve with sucking at the breast, the bottle feeds will be decreased.

Many premature babies take in more milk during some of their early breastfeeding by using a thin silicone nipple shield during the feeds. The shield holds the nipple out for the baby and can make it easier for him to take in the milk. A nipple shield can also be very useful when transitioning the baby from bottle to breast. Once this step is taken and the baby is latching on and nursing with the nipple shield, the next step is to wean from the shield and get the baby latching directly onto the breast. Beginning the feed with the nipple shield and taking it off about five minutes into the feed can do this. Usually the baby will latch onto the breast and continue nursing without the shield. If this does not work, go back to using the shield and try weaning from it again in a few days.

During this transition, Mum will still need to pump after the feed in order to remove milk from the breasts and stimulate the production of more. When the babies are feeding at least ten to twenty minutes on one or both breasts, with audible swallows at a ratio of one to two sucks followed by a swallow, they may not need additional pumped milk and

Mum may no longer need to pump after the feed. The other signs of good milk intake are six to eight wet nappies and about four stools a day.

Many mothers in my survey reported that even after bringing their premature twins home, weak sucking ability continued to be a complicating factor with breastfeeding. Here again is where a hospital-grade breast pump can be a huge help: pumping will help you keep your breast milk supply up, and feeding the twins breast milk from a bottle will reassure you that they are getting the nutrition they need. As they get older, their sucking ability and coordination *will improve*. Patience is key! Of course, regular GP visits – during which your twins will be weighed – will also reassure you that you are making progress.

> '*The advice I would give to mothers of premature twins is "Give breastfeeding a try, do it for as long as you can, as long as you are able to still enjoy other parts of your life . . . it is the hardest thing you will ever do, but if you do not succeed you are not a bad mother."*'

But what should you do when your babies are progressing at different rates? If one baby is feeding well at the breast and the other isn't, you should consider pumping the breast that has not been emptied well once the baby who is nursing poorly has stopped removing milk. This is a time when Dad or another helper may go ahead and feed a bottle of previously pumped milk or formula to the baby who needs a little more.

If you have got one twin breastfeeding directly and the other continuing to do some breastfeeding and some additional bottle-feeding, keeping a written record of what feeding method is used for each baby and how much milk is taken is essential. Although taking notes can seem tedious at times, knowing how much milk your babies are getting through bottle-feeding – and how much milk you are able to supply in a pump session – will give you the confidence to continue breastfeeding.

Regardless of your twins' breastfeeding prowess, some parents find that planning for one bottle-feed at night by Dad or another helper is good not only for milk production but for sanity as well! If Mum can get one four-to-six-hour stretch of sleep, she may find herself more rested and therefore better able to deal with breastfeeding during the day. If you try this system, Mum should pump before going to sleep and empty her breasts as fully as possible in order to encourage the development of a good milk supply. It might also be better for some mothers to supplement breastfeeding each twin with one bottle of pumped milk or formula a day. With this kind of regular break, many mums report, they have the emotional and physical stamina to continue breastfeeding; without that break, many mothers give up on breastfeeding altogether. Whatever you choose, don't beat yourself up or feel guilty! If your twins are continuing to grow and thrive – on breast milk, formula or a combination – you are doing well by them. Do what feels right and comfortable for you.

The Possible Effects of Assisted Reproductive Technology (ART)

There is some evidence that milk production may be lower among older first-time mothers and mothers who have had fertility treatments. A low milk supply is a difficult situation with one baby. When you have multiple babies and a low milk supply, it presents a bigger problem. We do know that some of the hormones important for mammary development are also important to the conception of a baby. These include prolactin, oestrogen, progesterone, thyroxine, insulin and cortisol. Having too much or too little of these hormones can affect breast milk production. Determining the reason for the infertility problem that required the intervention may also be helpful in solving the problem of low milk supply.

SUCCESS STORIES FROM NANCY NELSON, R.N., ICBLC

I have worked with countless breastfeeding mothers who have been able to breastfeed their twins and have easily – or eventually – been able to produce enough milk for them. There are so many variables with this issue that it is not simply a matter of supply and demand.

One mother I worked with did very well with breastfeeding her twins who were born at thirty-six weeks' gestation. She had used assisted reproduction therapy to get pregnant. She also had a two-year-old boy at home whom she had breastfed for nine months. In my experience, once a woman has breastfed one baby, it seems that the milk increases in volume more quickly after the delivery of the next baby or babies. Given that this mother had had the experience of handling a baby at the breast before, she felt more comfortable while breastfeeding her twins. She knew what signs to look for that would indicate that the babies were getting enough milk. She knew that producing six to eight urine nappies and four to six stools in a twenty-four-hour period was a great sign. The babies were feeding eight to twelve times in a twenty-four-hour period and were content between feeds. Recognising these factors helped her to relax more during the feeds, leading to a better 'let-down' reflex. This is the term that is used to describe the enlarging of the milk ducts that occurs as a result of the release of oxytocin (a hormone released by the pituitary gland) during breastfeeding.

Healthy let-down allows more milk to flow to the babies and, in this case, led to a stronger suck. In addition, this mother happened to have a great deal of help at home. Her husband and aunt were both there to help her for the first two months after she delivered the babies. She had taken out a loan so she could hire a baby nurse to come to her home at night and help her arrange a feeding plan, which allowed her to get some sleep at night. She told me that it was one of the best investments she had ever made.

If your twins are each producing six to eight wet (urine) nappies and four to six dirty (stool) nappies within a twenty-four-hour period, they are likely getting enough to eat.

Of course, you don't need to have had a singleton first to be able to produce milk and get the hang of breastfeeding quickly. I have worked with many mothers whose first pregnancy resulted in twins. Although it can sometimes take up to five days for milk to increase in volume after the babies are born, pumping and patience will quickly lead to success. You also don't need to hire help, but having support from your family – especially the father of the babies – is a tremendously important factor in breastfeeding successfully from the start.

Another woman I remember well was thirty-nine when she became a first-time mother of twins. She too had used ART to conceive her twins, and they were born at thirty-seven weeks. Because it made her feel more secure to know how much milk the babies were getting, she pumped with a hospital-grade pump from the time they were born and bottle-fed her babies with the expressed milk. In that way, she was able to produce enough milk for both of them.

When this mother brought her twins in for their two-month checkup, she asked me for help with engorgement, as her breasts were very full and hard. Though engorgement is usually a problem mainly when the milk first comes in right after babies are born, sometimes it occurs if feeds are missed.

At this two-month appointment, Mum did not have her pump with her, and so we decided to try to get one of the babies to latch on to help decrease the engorgement. The baby latched on almost immediately and nursed well for fifteen minutes!

This story illustrates what I have seen time and again: even after weeks of bottle-feeding, latch-on can occur. Mothers of preemies who have to bottle-feed initially should not feel that direct breastfeeding will never occur. I have seen babies as old as three months latch on and breastfeed after having been only bottle-fed.

BREASTFEEDING TWINS SIMULTANEOUSLY

Breastfeeding your twins simultaneously is time-efficient and will go a long way toward synchronising their eating and sleeping schedules right from the start. In the beginning, however, it may be a little difficult to breastfeed your twins simultaneously. They may have different sucking abilities, and simply holding more than one baby at the breast at a time is logistically a little complicated!

Many mothers start out by feeding the babies individually and gradually move on to feeding both babies at the same time. If you are feeding them separately, remember to alternate the breast you feed them with so that both breasts are emptied well, even if one of the babies has a weaker suck. Some mothers use the same breast for each baby for a twenty-four-hour period. Others alternate the breast they use for each baby every other feed.

There are two frequently used breastfeeding positions for feeding twins simultaneously: the double side hold and the double cradle hold. With the side hold, each baby is at your side with his or her feet extending behind you and supported by pillows. Bring each one to the breast he or she is facing. With the double cradle hold, each baby is in the crook of each arm in front of you, with their bodies crossing each other. Bring each baby to the breast he or she is facing. Use pillows to support the babies on your lap.

KEEPING UP YOUR MILK SUPPLY

The best recipe for successful breastfeeding is to establish a sufficient milk supply. When you have enough milk to satisfy your twins' needs, they'll nurse more comfortably and contentedly. If you don't have enough milk for both of them, they will be running on less nutrition than they need and be crankier and sleep less well as a result.

The key to keeping up your milk supply is to make sure that the milk is removed from your breasts on a regular basis, about every two to three hours around the clock, especially for the first two to three weeks after the babies are born. If your twins are premature or not sucking well, you can do this by pumping every two to three hours until they can breastfeed. If you're pumping to express your milk, you'll need to pump on each side for at least fifteen minutes with a hospital-grade pump (using a double pump helps to complete this process more quickly). Hospital-grade pumps can be rented through the NCT (see Resources), or various independent outlets online or from a private lactation consultant. Once your babies' sucking abilities have improved, you can return the rental pump and downgrade to a manual or battery-operated pump; however, you may discover that you need the more powerful pump to help you increase your milk supply as your twins have growth spurts and, in turn, increased nutritional needs.

> Many women find that putting warm compresses on their breasts while pumping or massaging their breasts while pumping greatly improves the let-down response and improves milk flow. Meditation and listening to relaxing music might also help to produce a stronger let-down, and ultimately a better milk supply.

Sufficient milk supply is also contingent on Mum taking care of herself! You need to be well nourished and hydrated to produce enough milk to satisfy your babies. Nancy and I recommend that new mums have six 'feeds' for themselves a day: breakfast, a mid-morning snack, lunch, a mid-afternoon snack, dinner and an evening snack. Have something to drink each time you breastfeed or pump. We also recommend lying down during the day and trying to get some rest while the babies are asleep or in the care of Dad or another helper. All of these things contribute to mothers being less stressed and ultimately having a better let-down, which should lead to a better milk supply.

In spite of doing these things, some mothers still have difficulty with producing enough milk for more than one baby. There is, of course, no magic pill you can take to increase your milk supply. You might hear that herbal supplements such as mother's milk tea and fenugreek will help your breast milk supply, but there is not sufficient research about the possible side effects of these supplements to recommend them.

Another thing you can do for yourself to support your desire to breastfeed is to establish a relationship with a lactation consultant during your pregnancy or early postpartum period. Your health visitor or GP should be able to point you in the direction of your local chapter of the La Leche League, a national organisation whose mission is to offer 'mother-to-mother support, encouragement, information and education to promote a better understanding of breastfeeding as an important element in the healthy development of the baby and mother'. Alternately, seek out (or start!) a mothers-of-multiples group in your area. In other mothers of twins you'll find support and the expertise that comes from personal experience.

As with sleeping schedules, writing down your breastfeeding schedule – what you hope to achieve each day as well as what actually happened – can help support your desire to breastfeed. Use a breastfeeding log (see Resources), and you'll be able to see your progress and see patterns emerging. Using a log will also help you keep things straight: which baby gets which breast when and which baby may be due for a bottle.

GO EASY ON YOURSELF!

Breastfeeding your twins is a wonderful gift to them and will provide you a natural and peaceful way to bond with each baby. But don't feel guilty if for some reason you cannot breastfeed exclusively. Some breastfeeding is better than no breastfeeding. And if you can't or choose not to breastfeed, there are many other aspects of good parenting that have nothing to do with feeding! Remember, you can be a loving parent when you are bathing, changing, talking and reading to, and simply playing with your children.

CHAPTER 7

Anticipating and Preparing for Possible Challenges with Sleep Training

Sleep-training twins is not a complicated process, but, as I have repeatedly stated throughout this book, there are many factors that will contribute to or detract from your likely success with it. To be sure, whether your twins are fraternal or identical can play a role in the logistics of sleep training, specifically how involved you might have to be in synchronising their schedules.

Who your twins are shaping up to be as individuals – their respective abilities to soothe themselves back to sleep, their tolerance for distraction and noise, and their own individual medical issues – will also certainly impact the process.

But as we've discussed throughout this book, who you are as parents – your age, your experience and what you might have been through to conceive your twins – can also influence when you initiate sleep training, how flexible or rigid you choose to be about it from the start and how you yourselves tolerate the process. For instance, whether you underwent assisted reproductive technology (ART) will, of course, influence the odds of your having fraternal or identical twins, but because of protracted attempts to have children this way, ART can also play a role in your mood and mind-set once the twins arrive. The wonderfully detailed narrative feedback from my surveys with more than a hundred sets of parents of twins bears this out clearly: what you bring to your role as parents will have an effect on your sleep-training experience. No two families are exactly alike, and what works for one family with a given certain set of circumstances may not work for another family with a similar background and set of circumstances. There is so much diversity among families of twins that you will have to adapt my sleep-training techniques and advice to work within *your* family and not rely exclusively on advice from another family with twins to guide you. Likewise, although the general advice given in this book applies to all twins, how each family implements it should be customised for its own circumstances.

That being said, my analysis of the feedback from parents of twins has led me to some observations about what contributes to the goal of having twins sleep well and what *might* make achieving that goal easier or more challenging for you. In this chapter I want to outline and summarise what I have observed so that you might be able to extrapolate from my findings and use my observations to inform the way you ready yourselves and customise the sleep-training process for your family. In talking with parents of twins, I also understand how much of a relief it can be for them to hear that they are not alone in the things that they find easy or difficult about this process. In sharing with you here the trends I have seen in working with parents of twins, I hope you also experience the relief that comes from knowing that you aren't the first to face these challenges.

> What I call 'challenging' elements *may* be no challenge for one family, minor speed bumps for another family and major roadblocks for yet another family. The reason why challenging elements affect each family differently is that each family has a different balance of strengths and weaknesses that contributes to helping twins sleep well. So the presence or absence of a single challenging element has to be viewed in the context of the complete picture: your individual family dynamics.

WHAT MY SURVEY SHOWS

There are a number of overarching factors associated with how all twins sleep. But I want to clearly state that these factors do not apply equally to some subgroups of twins. So first, let's look at twins in general and what their parents report anecdotally. Later in this chapter, we'll look at what the data show about certain subgroups of twins.

How Mum's Age Can Impact the Experience of Sleep Training

The median age of the mothers in my survey was thirty-four. When I say 'young mothers' I am referring to mothers thirty-four years old and younger; 'older mothers' are thirty-five and older. What's important to take from these observations is not so much that a mother's age impacts her children's sleep in any medical or genetic way but that it impacts her impression of their sleep, her tolerance of a lack of it and her experience of other circumstances such as postpartum depression and her interest in breast-feeding.

- Young mothers compared to older mothers were more likely to describe *both* twins as sleeping well, whether they had successfully sleep-trained them or not. From this I infer that the younger the mother (and/or parents), the more tolerance they had for – and the more patience they had with – sleep issues. This anecdotal finding may suggest that twins of younger mothers actually sleep more or sleep better, perhaps because sleep training was started earlier. Alternatively, it may suggest that when mothers are younger, they are less bothered by the twins' sleep issues. Of course, there is nothing you can do now about your age! But I do believe that knowing that younger mothers tend to have this sunnier outlook will help you interpret what others are saying better and, most important, beat yourself up *far less* now that you know that age can play a role in the way a mother describes her experience.
- Young mothers were more likely to try to help their twins learn to sleep at or before four months of age (post-due date).
- Young mothers were more likely to be successful at

breastfeeding and less likely to have baby blues/post-partum depression.

HOW DAD'S AGE CAN IMPACT THE EXPERIENCE OF SLEEP TRAINING

The median age of the fathers in my survey was 36.5 years old, so when I refer to 'young fathers' I am talking about men who are thirty-six and younger; 'older fathers' refers to fathers who are thirty-seven and older.

- Young fathers were more likely to be involved in helping the twins sleep than were older fathers.
- Young fathers reported that their attempts to help the twins sleep began before four months of age.
- Young fathers often had a child before the twins were born, and the presence of an older sibling is associated with parents describing the twins as *both* sleeping well.

HOW DAD'S INVOLVEMENT AT HOME CAN IMPACT SLEEP TRAINING

- In almost every survey, when fathers played an active role in caring for the twins and took part in sleep-training them, the sleep training went more smoothly and was successful at an earlier point in the process.
- If a father had children from another marriage previous to having twins or had been around for and helpful with an older sibling within the current marriage, mothers reported that he was more helpful and more active in the sleep-training process.

HOW BABY BLUES/POSTPARTUM DEPRESSION CAN IMPACT THE EXPERIENCE OF SLEEP TRAINING

- Mothers who reported having either baby blues or post-partum depression were generally less likely to describe *both* twins as sleeping well and were more likely to describe only *one* twin as sleeping well. It is not known what might come first: baby blues/postpartum depression interfering with sleep training or twins who have difficulty sleeping triggering baby blues or postpartum depression.

- Mothers with baby blues/postpartum depression were more likely to describe one of their twins as having colic, which made sleep training a little harder until the colic had passed.

- When mothers reported baby blues or postpartum depression, they also reported that the duration of breastfeeding was shorter than that of mothers who did not have baby blues or postpartum depression. Here again, it is not known what might come first: baby blues or postpartum depression interfering with breastfeeding or difficulties in breastfeeding triggering baby blues or postpartum depression.

HOW HAVING USED ASSISTED REPRODUCTIVE TECHNOLOGY (ART) CAN IMPACT THE EXPERIENCE OF SLEEP TRAINING

- The effect of ART on parenting is not the same for all mothers. Younger mothers, mothers with a shorter duration of infertility, mothers with fewer unsuccessful attempts at ART, mothers with no miscarriages or terminations following ART and mothers who already had a child were less inclined to attribute any effect of ART on parenting.

- Mothers who had more protracted or disappointing experiences with ART more often attributed an effect of ART on parenting that sometimes included a reluctance to initiate sleep training.
- ART is associated with more baby blues and postpartum depression.

HOW HAVING AN OLDER CHILD IN ADDITION TO TWINS CAN IMPACT THE EXPERIENCE OF SLEEP TRAINING

- Strict synchronised scheduling, starting early, was often used in order to have some predictable time with the twins' older sibling.
- Mothers of twins who had previously successfully breastfed a child reported having more confidence in their ability to breastfeed twins. They were more likely to breastfeed exclusively (rather than supplement with formula), but the duration of breastfeeding was shorter compared to families where there was no older sibling.
- Mothers who had a child before having the twins were more often than not older mothers and therefore often reported less energy to tolerate a lack of sleep. Maybe this translated into more motivation to sleep-train from an earlier date.
- Mothers who had a child before having the twins were less likely to have used ART, and they were less likely to experience baby blues or postpartum depression.

How Colic Can Impact the Experience of Sleep Training

- When a twin has colic, parents reported that the colicky twin did not sleep well.
- Colic is associated with baby blues or postpartum depression. This is not to suggest that a mother with postpartum depression or baby blues is more likely to have a colicky baby; rather, it suggests that colic is a difficult thing to contend with in the early months of a baby's or babies' lives and the stress that comes with dealing with it can trigger or exacerbate blues or depression in the new mother.
- The younger the gestational age at birth, the more colic was reported in my survey.

How Prematurity Can Impact the Experience of Sleep Training

- In addition to reporting more colic, parents of premature twins were more tentative with sleep training than those whose twins were born full term. Indeed, parents of premature twins generally reported delaying getting started with sleep training until their twins were more than four months old (post-due date).
- Complications of prematurity sometimes included difficulty in sucking and weight gain or the logistics of having one twin at home and the other twin in the NICU. But there were positive aspects reported as a result of prematurity: the twins got onto a regular schedule while in the hospital; the parents had more time to prepare for child care while the twins were in

the hospital; and parents enjoyed the one-on-one time with one twin at home if the other was still in the hospital. Your experiences and those of other parents of premature twins *might* be totally different because near-term premature twins (thirty-four to thirty-six weeks gestational age) are much more like term babies than very premature twins (thirty-three weeks and less gestational age).

How a Maternity Leave or a Return to Work for Mum Can Impact Sleep Training

- Mothers who had a short maternity leave (of no more than six weeks) reported starting to sleep-train early and being very strict about synchronised scheduling. Such strict scheduling permitted mothers to get some sleep for themselves before they returned to work.
- Mothers working outside the home sometimes felt guilty about spending less time with their twins during the day and compensated by keeping them up too late at night, which in turn created problems with healthy sleep in their twins.

The Specific Data on Groups of Twins

Above are the general and anecdotal results of my survey, but now let's look at the four distinct groups of twins that emerged as significant from my research. Specifically, in addition to whether twins were fraternal or identical, maternal age and reproductive history (whether or not Mum underwent ART) proved to be the factors most influencing sleep training.

Even though I hope it will be instructive and helpful to see what other people of your age and reproductive history have experienced, it bears repeating that no matter what group you are in, the differences described below are not your destiny! There are countless factors that cut across these groups and that might be unique to your situation. And remember, unlike the parents in my survey, you have benefited from reading this book and creating your own success story!

The four groups are:

A. Identical twins, no ART
B. Fraternal twins, no ART (the oldest mother was thirty-eight years old)
C. Fraternal twins, ART (the oldest mother was thirty-eight years old)
D. Fraternal twins, ART (the youngest mother was thirty-nine years old)

These four groups allow us to compare both the general experience of parenting twins and the specific impact of various factors on sleep and sleep training. We can see the differences between identical and fraternal twins (A versus B), no ART and ART (B versus C), and younger and older mothers (C versus D).

GROUP A VERSUS GROUP B: IDENTICAL COMPARED TO FRATERNAL TWINS

My comparison, based on data from the two groups, shows that:

- Among Identical Twins (no ART), *both* twins were more likely to sleep well and were less likely to have colic.

Mothers of identical twins were less likely to have baby blues/postpartum depression and were more likely to breastfeed even though they were older. This supports research showing that when mothers breastfeed and their babies sleep well, it is less likely that mothers will experience postpartum depression. However, in general, difficulties in breastfeeding and pastpartum depression are more likely among older mothers. Fathers of identical twins were more involved in helping twins sleep even though they were older. However, in general, my survey shows that older fathers provide less help in sleep-training twins.

GROUP B VERSUS GROUP C: NO ART COMPARED TO ART

My comparison, based on data from the two groups, shows that:

- Among Fraternal Twins (no ART), *both* twins were more likely to sleep well and less likely to have colic. They were more likely to have an older brother or sister, and in general, the presence of an older child made it more likely for both twins to sleep well.
- Mothers of Fraternal Twins (no ART) were less likely to have baby blues or postpartum depression (even though in my sampling these mothers were breastfeeding less). This supports the research showing that having twins after a period of infertility with ART increases psychological stress in mothers. However, in general, less breastfeeding is associated with more baby blues/

postpartum depression. Also, this supports the research showing that when children sleep better, it is less likely that the mothers will become depressed postpartum.

- Fathers of Fraternal Twins (no ART) were less involved in helping the twins sleep even though they were younger. However, in general, older fathers are less involved in helping with sleep-training the twins.

GROUP C VERSUS GROUP D: YOUNGER MOTHERS COMPARED TO OLDER MOTHERS

My comparison, based on data from the two groups, shows that:

- In the Fraternal Twins (ART), Younger Mothers group, *both* twins were more likely to sleep well and less likely to have colic. They were less likely to have an older brother or sister, but in general, the presence of an older child made it more likely for both the twins to sleep well. Younger mothers were less likely to have baby blues or postpartum depression and were more likely to breastfeed only. Surprisingly, as observed by Linda, all older mothers in this group reported having baby blues or postpartum depression, except those who were married to younger men.

- Younger fathers in the Fraternal Twins (ART), Younger Mothers group were more involved in helping the twins sleep. But it should be noted that some of the older fathers, including the oldest father (age sixty-four when the twins were born) had previous marriages with children, and in this subgroup of experienced fathers, they were very involved in caring for their twins. But in general, older fathers were less involved.

Now let's compare all four groups:

	Identical, No ART	Fraternal, No ART	Fraternal, ART, Younger Mothers	Fraternal, ART, Older Mothers
Both Twins Sleep Well	60%	33%	28%	22%
BB/PPD	13%	20%	40%	67%
Colic	9%	19%	32%	40%

Looking at these four groups from left to right, you can see that it becomes consistently less likely that both twins will sleep well and more likely that there will be baby blues/postpartum depression and colic to complicate the dynamics. These consistent trends across all four groups illustrate how different the journeys *might* be for different families of twins. When you add the likelihood of exclusively breastfeeding and having the father involved in helping with sleeping, you can see how the parents of Identical Twins (no ART) *might* have a much easier trip than those of Fraternal Twins (ART), Older Mothers.

	Identical, No ART	Fraternal, No ART	Fraternal, ART, Younger Mothers	Fraternal, ART, Older Mothers
Breastfeeding Only	73%	33%	39%	9%
Father's Involvement	92%	76%	88%	70%

I want to restate that though your place within one of these four different groups might resonate with your own experiences, the group you are in does *not* determine your destiny. Having read this book and learned about sleep training and its many benefits, you have the information and power to counterbalance any challenges your age or reproductive history *theoretically* predispose you to! Furthermore, if you reflect on how the more general circumstances discussed at the beginning of this chapter interact with the four different data groups – whether your twins were premature, whether you have another child or children in the family, whether you have to go back to work, etc. – it becomes clear that your approach to teaching your twins how to sleep can be tailored to fit the specific features of your family.

In the end, and despite all factors, the advice given by mothers in each of the four groups was exactly the same for three important questions.

Q: What was the most important factor for twins' sleep?

A: 'Schedules: Synchronise the sleep schedules from the start.'

Q: What was the most important factor in maintaining your sanity?

A: 'Synchronise the twins' schedules, and get help!'

Q: What was the most important factor in maintaining marital harmony?

A: 'Communicate – make a team.'

Resources

There is a lot of information in books and magazines and on the Internet related to twins. Rather than try to be exhaustive in listing everything, here are is a list of key resources.

Parenting Twins and General Health Information

BOOKS

A Contented House with Twins by Gina Ford and Alice Beer (Vermilion, 2006)

Twins and Multiple Births: The Essential Parenting Guide from Pregnancy to Adulthood by Carol Cooper (Vermilion, 2004)

WEBSITES

Directgov
Provides easy access to government information and

services, including those for parenting and healthcare.
www.direct.gov.uk

MBF (The Multiple Births Foundation)
An independent charity based at Queen Charlotte's &
Chelsea Hospital in West London. A vital resource to
professionals and families alike, it aims to improve the care
and support of multiple-birth families through the education
of all relevant professionals.
www.multiplebirths.org.uk

NCT (National Childbirth Trust)
The UK's leading charity for parents. They support people
through the life-changing experience of pregnancy, birth
and early parenthood, offering relevant information,
reassurance and mutual support.
www.nctpregnancyandbabycare.com

NHS Choices
Information from the National Health Service on conditions,
treatments, local services and healthy living.
www.nhs.uk

Sure Start
The UK government's programme to deliver the best start in
life for every child by bringing together early education,
childcare, health and family support.
www.dcsf.gov.uk/everychildmatters/about/surestart

Tamba (The Twins and Multiple Births Association)
A charity set up by parents of twins, triplets and higher
multiples and interested professionals.
www.tamba.org.uk

Prematurity
Bliss
This special care baby charity provides vital support and care
to premature and sick babies across the UK. They offer
guidance and information to families.
www.bliss.org.uk

Prematurity.org
A comprehensive US site devoted to information, other
recommended resources and support for parents of
premature babies.
www.prematurity.org

Feeding

BOOKS

Amy Spangler's Breastfeeding: A Parent's Guide by Amy Spangler
(Amy Spangler, 1999)

The Nursing Mother's Companion: Revised Edition by Kathleen
Higgins (Harvard Common Press, 2005)

*What to Expect When You're Breast-feeding . . . And What If You
Can't?* by Clare Byam-Cook (Vermilion, 2006)

WEBSITES

The Breastfeeding Network
An independent source of support and information for breastfeeding women and those involved in their care.
www.breastfeedingnetwork.org.uk

La Leche League
An organisation that aims to help mothers to breastfeed through mother-to-mother support, encouragement, information and education.
www.laleche.org.uk

Postpartum Depression
NHS Choices: Postnatal Depression
The NHS information page about this condition.
www.nhs.uk/conditions/postnataldepression/pages/introduction.aspx

Postpartum Support International
An organisation dedicated to helping women suffering from perinatal mood and anxiety disorders, including postpartum depression.
www.postpartum.net

Royal College of Psychiatrists
This website has a page dedicated to postnatal depression with information and advice for sufferers, family and friends.
www.rcpsych.ac.uk/mentalhealthinfo/problems/
postnatalmentalhealth/postnataldepression.aspx

Colic

BOOKS

Coping with Crying and Colic by Siobhan Mulholland (Vermilion, 2008)

Your Fussy Baby by Dr Marc Weissbluth (Ballantine Books, 2003)

WEBSITES

NHS Choices: Colic
The NHS information page about this condition.
www.nhs.uk/conditions/colic/pages/introduction.aspx

Tracking Feeding and Sleeping

BOOKS

The Essential Breastfeeding Log by Suzanne Schlosberg and Sarah Bowen Shea (Ballantine Books, 2009)

WEBSITES

Babycenter: How to Track Your Baby's Sleeping Patterns
This US website offers a downloadable blank chart to help you track hours of sleep.
www.babycenter.com/0_how-to-track-your-babys-sleeping-patterns_7643.bc

Acknowledgements

I wish to thank all the parents of multiples who took time out from their hectic lives to answer my survey. Their thoughtful narrative responses provided the raw data for this book because there is no previously published information on sleep-training twins. I spent many hours analysing the survey responses to see if there were differences between identical versus fraternal twins born without or with assisted reproductive technology, breastfeeding versus formula feeding, younger versus older mothers, colic versus no colic, and many other variables. For her patience with me during those long days and nights of data analysis, I thank my wife, Linda.

As a clinical investigator, I felt obliged to present all of the findings, but as a practising paediatrician I knew that I had to translate the raw material into useful advice for tired parents of twins. General conclusions emerged from my analyses, but there was too much information to easily digest. Enter my editor, Marnie Cochran.

Marnie succinctly summarised an enormous amount of material to achieve more focus and clarity, reorganised the material so a tired parent could quickly be helped without feeling lost and encouraged me to maintain an optimistic tone throughout the book so a parent with the possible challenges of helping twins sleep better would not be discouraged. Thank you, Marnie, for your creative and skilful guidance.

I also wish to thank Nancy Nelson for giving us her words of wisdom and encouragement on breastfeeding twins despite the possibly formidable challenges of prematurity.

Index

academic performance, 9
activity, decreased, 39
adenoids, 25
afternoon nap, 23, 103–104,
    109, 111
age groups, 16, 17, 85–119
    duration of sleep and, 18–22,
        85–119
    four to eight weeks, 92–96
    four to six months, 104–107
    newborns, 87–92
    nine to twelve months,
        111–13
    nine to twelve weeks,
        96–100
    one to two years, 113–15
    six to nine months,
        108–111
    thirteen to sixteen weeks,
        100–104
    three to four years, 117–19
    two to three years, 115–17
aggression, 9

air travel, 8
American Academy of
    Pediatrics, 45, 155
anger, 9
assisted reproductive technology
    (ART), xi–xii, 76, 131,
        139–40
    breastfeeding and, 131, 132,
        133
    data on, 147–52
    effects on parenting, 76, 140,
        144–45, 147–52
    sleep training and, 144–45,
        147–52
athletics, 9

baby blues, x, xii, 7, 84, 143,
    145, 146, 149
    data on, 147–52
    effect on sleep-training
        experience, 144, 147–52
babysitters, 35, 52, 56, 67
baths, 45, 47–48, 107

bed, 117
  family, 44, 45
  transition from cot to,
    117–18
bedtime, *see* night
biological necessity of sleep, 6
biological sleep rhythms, 27–28,
    37, 72, 88, 92, 97
blanket, warm, 47
blood pressure, high, 7, 10
body aches, 5
body temperature, 18, 27, 28
books, 155–59
bottle-feeding, 19, 51, 74, 92
  father and, 74, 129–30
  premature twins, 128, 129,
    130, 134
  slower sucking, 39
boys, 14
brain, 9, 10–12, 16
  development, and sleep,
    10–12, 19, 52, 89, 97
  poor sleep and, 9
breastfeeding, 14, 19, 51, 60,
    64, 71, 74, 92, 123–38,
    142, 149, 152
  age of mother and, 143
  assisted reproductive
    technology and, 131, 132,
    133
  hormones and, 131, 132,
    137

keeping up milk supply,
    135–38
log, 138, 159
low milk production, 131
older child, 145
positions, 135
postpartum depression and,
    144
premature twins, 123–24,
    125–30, 135–36
pumping milk, 127–30,
    133–34, 135–36
resources, 159
slower sucking, 39
as soothing behaviour, 60, 64,
    73–74
success stories, 131–34
transition from bottle to
    breast, 128–29, 134
twins simultaneously,
    134–35

Caesarean delivery, 8, 124
California, 85
calmness, 39, 111
check and console strategy,
    58, 65
Chicago, 85
circadian timing system, 18
climbing out of cot, 116
cognitive development, 10–12,
    19, 52, 89, 97

colds, 116–17

colic, 8, 20, 21, 44, 60, 80, 84, 90–91, 102, 144, 146
  four to eight weeks old, 94–96
  impact on sleep-training experience, 146–52
  resources, 159

communication, parental, 69, 70, 153

computers, 86, 155

consolidation, sleep, 16, 25–26, 73

controlled crying (graduated extinction), 59–60, 65

cortisol, 12, 23, 27, 131

cosleeper, 45

cot, 44
  climbing out of, 116
  in separate rooms, 116
  tents, 116
  transition to bed from, 117–18

crankiness, *see* fussiness; irritability

crib, 43–45, 61
  same vs. separate, for twins, 43–44, 58, 79, 91, 92
  in separate rooms, 63–64

crying, 5, 14, 20, 29, 39, 56–65, 78, 106, 107
  check and console, 58, 65

controlled (graduated extinction), 59–60, 65

crying it out (extinction), 60–65

dealing with, 57–65

four to eight weeks old, 94–96

newborn's, 90–92

of one twin, and effect on the other, 57, 61, 63, 79, 91, 92, 94, 95

parental tolerance for, 57, 64, 73

sleep log, 80–83

sleep training and, 56–65

crying it out (extinction), 60–65

day care, 30, 106

Dement, William C., 10

depression, *see* baby blues; postpartum depression

diabetes, 9, 10

distractions, shutting out, 49

double duty, one parent pulling, 106–107

drowsiness, 37–40, 45, 58
  in controlled crying strategy, 59, 60
  putting twins down to sleep drowsy but awake, 37–40
  signals, 39–40, 54, 58, 60, 78, 85, 89, 95, 97, 98

drowsiness (*cont'd*)
  sleep routines and, 45, 48–49
due date, 17, 89
duration of sleep, 16, 18–22,
    85–119
  four to eight weeks old, 92–96
  four to six months old,
    104–107
  newborns, 87–92
  nine to twelve months old,
    111–13
  nine to twelve weeks old,
    96–100
  one to two years old, 113–15
  six to nine months old,
    108–111
  thirteen to sixteen weeks old,
    100–104
  three to four weeks old,
    117–19
  two to three years old, 115–17
dummy, 46–47

early evening, 5
  as witching hour, 105–106,
    115
England, 85
exhaustion, 9, 13
extinction, 60–65
eye contact, breaking, 40
eyes:
  drooping eyelids, 40, 97
    less visual focus, 40
  rubbing, 40, 97

family, 3–15, 140–41
  anticipating and preparing
    for challenges with sleep
    training, 139–53
  bed, 44, 45
  diversity, 140
  importance of sleep for,
    3–15
  See also father; grandparents;
    marriage; mother; parents;
    siblings
father, x, 6, 48
  age of, and effect on sleep
    training, 143, 149, 150
  at bedtime, 73–76
  bottle-feeding and, 74,
    129–30
  involvement at home, 143
  sleep-training role, 66–76,
    91–92, 143, 149–52
  soothing by, 60, 64, 73–76
  See also parents
feeding, 9, 58
  breastfeeding challenges and
    tips, 123–38
  charts, 80–81
  four to six months old, 105
  newborns, 87, 89–90, 92
  resources, 157, 159

synchronised schedules,
50–52, 53, 89–90
See also bottle-feeding;
breastfeeding
flexibility, importance of, 107
formula, *see* bottle-feeding
Foundation for the Study of
Infant Deaths (FSID), 44,
45
four to eight weeks old, 17, 19,
21, 27, 37, 40, 52, 59,
92–96
crying and colic, 94–96
duration of sleep, 92–96
four to six months old, 19, 22,
23, 104–107
crying it out (extinction),
60–65
duration of sleep,
104–107
witching hour, 105–106
fragmented sleep, 25–26
fraternal twins, xi, 13, 42, 50,
79, 139, 140
data on, 147–52
sleep patterns in, 88, 97, 102,
110, 114, 147–52
free time, of parents, 55–56,
95–96
fundamentals, sleep, xii–xiii,
1–31
brain development and, 10–12

consolidated sleep, 25–26
definition of healthy sleep,
16–31
duration of sleep, 18–22
effects of sleep deprivation,
6–8, 12
importance for whole family,
3–15
naps, 22–24
regularity of sleep, 30–31
sleep begets sleep, 12–13
sleep quality, 9–10
sleep schedules and timing of
sleep, 26–30
slight sleep loss, 4–6
twins as individuals, 13–15
fussiness, 9, 14, 20, 40, 41, 77,
90, 106
four to eight weeks old, 94–96
newborn's, 90–92
of one twin, and effect on the
other, 57, 61, 63, 79, 91,
92, 94, 95

gastrointestinal oesophageal
reflux disorder (GORD), 8,
20, 36, 44, 51, 80, 84, 90,
123–24
genetics, 18, 23, 88, 115
gentle pressure, 46
germs, 116
girls, 14

glucose control, impaired, 10
graduated extinction, 59–60, 65
grandparents, 35, 52, 77–79,
    91, 114
Guilleminault, Christian, 10

hand-eye coordination, 9
headaches, 5, 7, 28, 41
health information, general,
    155–57
health visitor, 45, 51, 87,137
healthy sleep, 16–31
    definition of, 16–31
Healthy Sleep Habits, Happy Child
    (Weissbluth), x
heart rate, 7
herbal supplements, 137
high blood pressure, 7, 10
homeostatic control
    mechanism, 17–18
hormones, 20–21
    breastfeeding and, 131, 132,
        137
    stress, 10, 12, 23, 27
    See also specific hormones
hospital, premature twins in,
    126–28, 146–47
hyperactivity, 9, 11

identical twins, xi, 13, 50, 79,
    139, 140
    data on, 147–52

sleep patterns in, 88, 102,
    115, 147–52
illness, 53, 80, 125
    premature babies and,
        125–26
    sleep setbacks and, 116–17
    at two to three years old,
        116–17
individuality of twins, 13–15,
    139
inflammation, 10
insulin, 131
Internet, 155–59
interruptions, sleep, 25–26
irritability, 9, 40, 96, 106, 115.
    See also fussiness

Japan, 85
jet lag, 28
junk food, 9
junk sleep, 9–10

lactation, *see* breastfeeding
lactation consultant, 137
La Leche League, 137, 157
let-down reflex, 132, 136
light-dark cycle, 18
log, sleep, 80–83

marriage, x, 100
    effect of sleep deprivation
        on, 7

sleep-training teamwork in,
67–76
See also father; mother;
parents
massage, 46
maternity leave, 147
maternity nurse, 38, 67, 77–79,
91
melatonin, 20–21, 27–28
midday nap, 101–102, 105,
108–109, 110, 111–12,
113, 113, 115–16
Minnesota, 85
modified extinction, 62–63
mood, 5
impaired, 9, 11, 25
morning nap, 23, 55, 101, 102,
105, 108–110, 111–12,
113, 114
mother, xii, 6, 48, 95
age of, and effect on sleep
training, 141–43, 147–53
assisted reproductive
technology and, 76, 140,
144–45, 147–52
breastfeeding, 123–38
crying twins and, 60–65
father as soother instead of,
60, 64, 73–76
free time of, 55–56, 95–96
postpartum depression and,
x, xii, 7, 84, 137, 142,

143, 144, 145, 146,
147–52
return to work, 106, 147
sleep-deprived, 6–8, 66, 80,
124
sleep-training role, 66–72,
91, 147–52
smell of, 58, 64, 74
voice of, 47
See also parents
'motion' sleep, 25
multitasking, 9
muscles, 20
aches, 41
strength, 11
tension, 7

nannies, 38, 52
nappy changes, 87, 129, 133
naps, 5, 12, 16, 22–24, 29, 37,
61, 73, 93
afternoon, 23, 103–104, 109,
111
brief intervals of wakefulness
between, in young babies,
40–45
four to six months old,
104–105
long, 24
midday, 101–102, 105,
108–109, 110, 111–112,
113, 114, 115–16

naps (*cont'd*)
  morning, 23, 55, 101, 102, 105, 108–110, 111–12, 113, 114
  nine to twelve months old, 111–12
  one to two years old, 113–15
  short, 24
  six to nine months old, 108–110
  stopping, 117
  synchronised sleep schedules, 52–56, 102, 110
  third, 103–104, 109, 111
  thirteen to sixteen weeks old, 100–104
  three to four years old, 117–118
  transition from two to one, 114–15
  two to three years old, 115–16
Nelson, Nancy, 123, 131
neonatal intensive care unit (NICU), 126–28, 146
newborns, 19, 36, 37, 40, 49, 87–92
  crying, 90–92
  duration of sleep, 87–92
  feeding, 87, 89–90, 92
  synchronising, 89–90
night, 29, 30, 31, 73, 93
  dads at bedtime, 73–76

four to eight weeks old, 92–93
four to six months old, 105–107
nine to twelve months old, 111–12
nine to twelve weeks old, 96–100
one parent pulling double duty at, 106–107
one to two years old, 114
six to nine months old, 109
sleeping schedules, 52–56
'sleeping through the', 21–22
thirteen to sixteen weeks old, 100, 102, 103
three to four years old, 117–18
two to three years old, 116–17
waking, 26, 64, 105, 112
nine to twelve months old, 17, 23, 111–13
  duration of sleep, 111–13
  naps, 111–12
nine to twelve weeks old, 17, 19, 37, 40, 52, 96–100
  duration of sleep, 96–100
  earlier bedtimes, 98, 99–100
nipple shield, 128

obesity, 9, 10
oestrogen, 131

older child, 55, 84, 143,
145
sleep-training twins and, 145
one to three weeks old, *see*
newborns
one to two years old, 17, 23,
113–15
duration of sleep, 113–15
transition from two naps to
one, 114–15
optimal wakefulness, 11–12,
13, 22
overtiredness, 29, 40, 41, 49,
58, 97, 98, 106
signs of, 40, 106
witching hour, 105–106
oxytocin, 132

parents, x–xi, 139–40
age of, xi, 141–43, 147–52
anticipating and preparing
for challenges with sleep
training, 139–53
communication between, 69,
70, 153
'free time' of, 55–56
one parent pulling double
duty, 106–107
premature babies and,
125–30
resources for, 155–57
roles of, 70–76

sleep deprived, 6–8, 66, 80
as sleep-training team,
67–76, 80–84
soothing by, 37, 38, 45–49,
58, 59–60, 64, 73–76, 80,
107, 111
See also father; mother
patience, 67, 142
persistence, 26
personality, impaired, 9
pituitary gland, 137
play, 111
calm vs. animated, 111
postpartum depression, x, xii, 7,
84, 137, 142, 143, 145,
146
breastfeeding and, 144
data on, 147–52
effect on sleep training, 144,
147–52
resources, 158
premature twins, 8, 21, 36, 50,
80, 84, 87, 90, 113,
123–24, 146–47
bottle-feeding, 128, 129, 130,
134
breastfeeding, 123–24,
125–30, 135–36
duration of sleep and, 88, 89
impact on experience of
sleep training, 146–47
resources on, 157

premature twins (*cont'd*)
  slightly vs. very premature,
    125
progesterone, 131
prolactin, 131, 137
pumped milk, 127–30, 133–34,
    135–36

quality, sleep, 9–10
quietness, 39

rapid eye movement (REM), 23
regularity, sleep, 16, 30–31
resources, 155–59
rhythmic motions, 46
rhythms, sleep, *see* biological
    sleep rhythms
routines, sleep, 45–49
  protecting, 49
rules, sleep, 118–19

schedules, 16, 26–30, 50–56
  adjusted for special occasions,
    112–13
  feeding, 50–52, 89–90
  night and nap sleep, 52–56
  synchronised, 50–56, 57,
    89–90, 102, 110, 134, 153
second wind, 12–13, 98, 106
self-agency, 110–11
self-soothing, 36–37, 38, 42, 57,
    90, 91–92

depriving opportunities
    for, 38
separate rooms, 63–64, 116
siblings, 55
  fussing of, 57, 61, 63, 79, 91,
    92, 94, 95
  older, 55, 84, 143, 145
signals:
  drowsiness, 39–40, 54, 58,
    60, 78, 85, 89, 95, 97, 98
  sleep, 29
singing, 47
six to nine months old, 17, 23,
    108–111
  duration of sleep, 108–111
  naps, 108–111
  self-agency, 110–11
Sleep, 10
sleep/wake pattern, 27, 28
sleep deprivation, 4–6, 41, 61,
    65, 66, 80, 103, 106
  effects of, 6–8, 12, 124
  premature babies and, 126,
    127
  slight, 4–6
sleeping arrangements, 43–45
'sleeping through the night',
    meaning of, 21–22
sleep training, x, 35–65
  age groups and, 85–119
  age of mother and, 141–43,
    147–52

anticipating and preparing
for challenges with, 139–53
brief intervals of wakefulness
between frequent naps,
40–45
crying and, 56–65
five steps, 37–65
log, 80–83
putting twins down to sleep
drowsy but awake, 37–40
soothing sleep routines,
45–49
synchronized schedules,
50–56, 57, 89–90, 102,
110, 134, 153
team, 66–84
troubleshooting, 121–53
when to start, 36–37
slower motions, 39
smiles, 20, 96
soothing:
breastfeeding as, 60, 64,
73–74
by maternity nurse or
grandparents, 77–79
by parents, 37, 38, 45–49, 58,
59–60, 64, 73–76, 80, 107,
111
self-, 36–37, 38, 42, 57, 90,
91–92
sleep log, 80–83
sleep routines, 45–49

techniques, 46–48
sounds, 47
special occasions, and sleep
schedule, 112–13
stomach aches, 28
stool, 133
strategies, sleep, 33–119
children's sleep needs at
different ages, 85–119
sleep-training team, 66–84
sleep-training twins, 35–65
stress, 7, 71
hormones, 10, 12, 23, 27
success stories, breastfeeding,
131–34
sucking, 46–47, 90, 123, 132
in premature babies, 123,
127–28, 129, 135–36, 146
summer, 117
sympathetic nervous system,
12
synchronised schedules, 50–56,
57, 89–90, 102, 110, 134,
153

team, sleep-training, 66–84
dads at bedtime, 73–76
maternity nurse, 77–79
parents as, 67–76, 80–84
right kind of help, 77–79
roles, 70–76
sleep log, 80–83

teething, 5

television, 86

temperature, body, 18, 27, 28

thirteen to sixteen weeks old,
17, 19, 22, 40, 52, 60,
100–104

  crying it out (extinction),
60–65

  duration of sleep, 100–104

  midday nap, 101–102

  morning nap, 101

  third nap, 103–104

three to four years old, 17,
117–19

  duration of sleep, 117–19

  'sleep rules,' 118–19

thumb sucking, 47

thyroxine, 131

timing of sleep, 16, 26–30

tonsils, 25

total sleep hours, 85–86

troubleshooting, 121–53

  anticipating and preparing
for challenges with sleep

  training, 139–53

  breastfeeding challenges and
tips, 123–38

two to three years old, 115–17

  climbing out of cot, 116

  duration of sleep, 115–17

  illness, 116–17

urination, 133

vocalisation, less, 39

wave, sleep, 29–30

websites, 155–59

weight, 52, 89

  birth, 52, 53

  gain, 50–51, 52, 129, 146

  sleep rhythms and, 89

  twins with different
weights, 89

wind, 5, 90–91. *See also* colic

witching hour, 105–106, 115

work, 106

  return to, 106, 147

ABOUT THE AUTHOR

Married to his wife, Linda, for forty-four years, Dr Marc Weissbluth has been a paediatrician for more than thirty-five years. A leading researcher on sleep and children, he founded the original Sleep Disorders Center at Children's Memorial Hospital in Chicago and is a professor of clinical paediatrics at the Northwestern University School of Medicine. Dr Weissbluth discovered that sleep is linked to temperament and that sleeping problems are related to infant colic, and he coined the now-familiar phrase 'sleep training' to describe his method for helping children fall asleep. His finding that changing the time a child is put to bed dramatically decreases the number of night awakenings was published in the prestigious journal *Sleep* in 1982. His landmark seven-year study on the development and disappearance of naps highlighted the importance of daytime sleep. In addition to his own research, he has written chapters on sleep problems in textbooks for paediatricians, lectured extensively to parent groups and appeared on *The Oprah Winfrey Show*. Dr Weissbluth is the father of four sons and six grandchildren – and they are all good sleepers. Dr and Mrs Weissbluth live in Chicago.

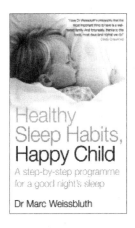